GLYCEMIC COUNTER

Dr. Wynnie Chan

GLYCEMIC INDEX & GLYCEMIC LOAD RATINGS

COMPLETE NUTRITIONAL FACTS FOR EVERY DIET

NEW EDITION

The majority of the nutrient information has been calculated using data from the UK Food Nutrient Databank which is available from The Food Standards Agency (FSA). Some values have been either estimated based on similar foods or obtained from relevant manufacturers. The Chinese dim sum values from been obtained from the Department of Health in Hong Kong.

The information in this book is intended only as a guide to following a healthy diet. People with special dietary requirements of any kind should consult appropriate medical professionals before changing their diet

An Hachette UK Company

www.hachette.co.uk

First published in Great Britain in 2006 by Hamlyn,

a division of Octopus Publishing Group Ltd

Endeavour House, 189 Shaftesbury Avenue, London, WC2H 8JY

www.octopusbooksusa.com

This edition published in 2014

Some of this material was previously published as Calorie Counter

Distributed in the US by Hachette Book Group USA

237 Park Avenue, New York NY 10017 USA

Distributed in Canada by Canadian Manda Group

165 Dufferin Street, Toronto, Ontario, Canada M6K 3H6

ISBN 978-0-600-62977-1

Printed and bound in China

10 9 8 7 6 5 4 3 2 1

What are GI and GL?

Glycemic index

The glycemic index (GI) is a measure of the ability of a food to raise blood glucose (sugar) levels after it has been eaten. The GI of a food is determined by several factors such as how much it's been processed, what type of cooking method has been used, and the presence of nutrients such as protein and fat.

How does it work?

When glucose is released into the bloodstream during digestion, our body produces a hormone called insulin, whose function is to transport glucose to places where it is needed for fuel—usually the muscle cells and the brain.

While our bodies can handle a steady release of glucose during digestion, when large quantities flood the bloodstream, the body's regulatory system goes into overload and produces large amounts of insulin to clear the glucose away into the body cells. This surge in insulin has the unfortunate effect of heightening our feelings of hunger, which in turn increases our desire to eat more carbs.

Regrettably, excess carbs get stored away in our fat cells. If this happens frequently, it can lead to weight gain and, over time, can even damage our cells by causing insulin resistance, where cells that normally respond to insulin become less sensitive to its effects.

Insulin resistance, high insulin levels, and excess high GI foods have all been linked with type 2, or middle-age onset, diabetes as well as premature aging, heart disease, and some cancers.

The benefits of eating low GI foods

Health experts believe that eating foods that cause a slow and steady rise of blood sugar levels, known as low GI foods, can have advantages for those watching their waistlines as well as for diabetic patients. This is because low GI foods help to delay feelings of hunger, compared to high GI foods, thus helping you to control your calorie intake.

There are a number of scientific studies that show that people who eat low GI foods lose more body fat than those who eat high GI foods.

Glycemic load

The glycemic load (GL) is a related measure and is calculated by multiplying the GI of a food by the amount of carbohydrate per typical serving and dividing it by 100.

GL is more reliable than the glycemic index as a predictor of how a food will affect the blood sugar level. This is because some foods that have a high GI, such as carrots or watermelon, contain such a small amount of carbohydrate in a normal portion that they would not be expected to raise the blood sugar levels much.

On the other hand, watermelon or carrot juice contains a larger amount of carbohydrate, which would cause a larger increase in blood sugar levels.

Glycemic load can be calculated using the following equation:

$$GL = \frac{GI \times carbohydrate\ per\ portion}{100}$$

New evidence is emerging that links high GL meals with an increased risk for heart disease and diabetes, especially in overweight and insulin-resistant people.

Understanding GI and GL ratings

- **Low GI and low GL** A food that has a low glycemic load will have a small effect on blood glucose levels, because it either doesn't contain a lot of carbohydrate and/or it has a low GI score.
- **Low GI and high GL** Even low GI foods, if eaten in large quantities, can affect (raise) blood glucose levels quite significantly, especially if they are concentrated sources of carbohydrates (for example, most cakes, dried fruit and dried fruit bars, fruit juices, and potato chips).
- **High GI and low GL** These foods contain a small amount of carbohydrate in typical serving sizes and will not affect blood glucose levels significantly even though they have a high GI. It is important to remember that these should not be eaten with other high GI or high GL foods.
- **High GI and high GL** These foods will cause a dramatic increase in blood glucose levels and so should be avoided wherever possible.

Healthy eating

Whether you want to lose just a few pounds or a lot more, eating healthily is vital. This does not mean cutting out all of your favorite treats completely, just eating them in moderation. If you're not enjoying your food, you probably won't follow your diet and exercise program.

Losing weight doesn't just mean that you'll have more energy and will feel better about yourself; it also decreases the risk of developing various ailments, including diabetes, hypertension, coronary heart disease, stroke, respiratory problems, gallstones, and some cancers.

A balanced diet

Including foods from the five food groups means that you are meeting your requirements for nutrients.

THE FIVE GROUPS ARE:
1 Bread, cereals, and potatoes This group is rich in starchy carbohydrates and includes breakfast cereals, rice, pasta, noodles, yams, and oats, and it should form the basis of most meals. Foods in this group are rich in insoluble fiber, calcium, iron, and the B vitamins, which are needed to keep your digestive tract, bones, and blood healthy. Try to eat whole-grain, whole-wheat or high-fiber versions of breads and cereals.

2 Fruits and vegetables These are important sources of antioxidants, such as vitamin C and beta-carotene (vegetable vitamin A), which protect us from cancers and heart disease. They are also rich in soluble fiber, which helps lower blood cholesterol. Try to include five portions of different fruits and vegetables in your diet each day, whether fresh, frozen, canned, dried, or juiced.

3 Milk and dairy foods These are excellent sources of calcium, protein, and vitamins A and B12, and they are essential for maintaining the health of bones, skin, and blood. Include a couple of reduced-fat servings from this food group each day.

4 Meat, fish, and alternatives The main nutrients supplied by this food group include iron, protein, the B vitamins, zinc, and magnesium, which help to maintain healthy blood and an efficient immune system. Daily, choose at most two servings of lean red meat, fish, chicken, nuts, turkey, eggs, and beans or other legumes. The last two are great protein alternatives to meat, as is tofu, which is also a good source of calcium.

5 Foods containing sugar or fat Minimize your intake of savory snacks, cookies, cakes, potato chips, pastries, candies, chocolate, pies, butter, and carbonated drinks, because these will hinder your efforts to lose weight.

How to use this book

This book lists the GI and GL rating, energy—as calories (cal) and joules (J)—fat, saturated fat, protein, carbohydrate, and fiber contained in more than 1,500 foods. Nutrient values have been expressed as average servings so no calculator is needed.

The information shows where the energy comes from in any food, so if you're on a low-carbohydrate, low-fat diet or have any other special requirements, you can work out exactly how much you can have of any food.

Recommended Daily Allowances

Recommended Daily Allowances (RDAs) are daily guideline figures recommended by health professionals for intake of calories, fat, and saturates for adult women and men. These are average figures and personal requirements will vary with age, weight, and levels of activity.

AVERAGE DAILY REQUIREMENT

	women	men
cal	2000	2500
fat	65g	80g
saturates	20g	25g

Dietary Reference Intakes

Dietary Reference Intakes (DRIs) are daily recommendations given by the U.S. Department of Agriculture (USDA) for the nutrients considered sufficient for most people in the United States. The table below gives the average daily requirement for protein, carbohydrate, and fiber. If you are trying to lose weight, you will need less, and should discuss the exact amounts with your physician or dietitian.

AVERAGE DAILY REQUIREMENT

	women	men
protein	46g	56g
carbohydrate	300g	375g
fiber	25g	25g

GI and GL ratings

Each food has been assigned a low, medium, or high GI and a low, medium, or high GL rating. The ratings are:

H = high
M = medium
L = low

FRUITS	AVERAGE PORTION oz	GI	GL
Apples, cooking	4.5	L	L
Apples, cooking, stewed with sugar	3.8	M	M
Apples, cooking, stewed without sugar	5	L	L
Apples, eating	3.5	L	L
Apricots	2.8	M	M
Apricots, canned in juice	5	M	M
Apricots, dried	4.2	L	L
Apricots, stewed with sugar	5	M	M
Apricots, stewed without sugar	5	L	L
Avocado	5.2	L	L
Banana chips	0.5	M	H
Bananas	3.5	M	M
Bilberries	1.4	L	L
Blackberries	3.5	L	L
Blackberries, stewed with sugar	5	M	M
Blackberries, stewed without sugar	5	L	L
Blackcurrants	3.5	L	L
Blackcurrants, canned in juice	5	M	M
Blackcurrants, canned in syrup	5	M	M
Blackcurrants, stewed with sugar	5	M	M
Blackcurrants, stewed without sugar	5	L	L
Blueberries	3.5	L	L
Cape gooseberry	2	L	L
Carambola	4.2	L	L
Cherries	2.8	L	L
Cherries, canned in syrup	2.4	M	M
Cherries, glacé	0.5	M	M
Clementines	2	L	L
Cranberries	2.6	L	L
Currants	0.8	H	H
Custard apples	2	L	L
Damsons	2.8	L	L
Damsons, stewed with sugar	3.5	M	M
Damsons, stewed without sugar	3.5	L	L

Unless otherwise stated, fruits are prepared but uncooked.

ENERGY cal	ENERGY J	FAT g	SATURATED FAT g	PROTEIN g	CARBO-HYDRATE g	FIBER g
46	196	Trace	Trace	0	12	2.1
81	345	Trace	Trace	0	21	1.3
56	237	0.4	0.1	0.3	13.6	1.8
51	215	0.5	0.1	0.6	11.6	1.3
25	107	Trace	Trace	1	6	1.4
48	206	Trace	Trace	1	12	1.3
190	809	1	Trace	5	44	7.6
101	431	Trace	Trace	1	26	2.2
38	161	Trace	Trace	1	9	2.1
276	1137	28.3	5.9	2.8	2.8	4.9
66	278	4	Trace	0	8	0.2
81	348	0.1	0	1.2	20.3	0.8
12	51	Trace	Trace	0	3	0.7
25	104	Trace	Trace	1	5	3.1
78	335	Trace	Trace	1	19	3.4
29	123	Trace	Trace	1	6	3.6
28	121	Trace	Trace	1	7	3.6
43	189	Trace	Trace	1	11	4.3
101	428	Trace	Trace	1	26	3.6
81	353	Trace	Trace	1	21	3.9
34	144	Trace	Trace	1	8	4.3
40	169	0.2	0	0.9	9.1	1.5
32	131	Trace	Trace	1	7	1
38	163	1	0.1	1	9	1.6
38	162	Trace	Trace	1	9	0.7
48	207	Trace	Trace	0	13	0.4
39	159	Trace	Trace	0	9	0
22	95	Trace	Trace	1	5	0.7
11	49	Trace	Trace	0	3	2.3
67	285	Trace	Trace	1	17	0.5
41	178	Trace	Trace	1	10	1.4
30	130	Trace	Trace	0	8	1.4
74	316	Trace	Trace	0	19	1.5
34	147	Trace	Trace	1	9	1.6

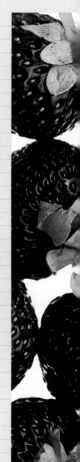

FRUITS	AVERAGE PORTION oz	GI	GL
Dates	3.5	H	H
Dates, stoned and dried	2	H	H
Durian	2.8	L	L
Figs	1.9	L	L
Figs, dried	3	H	H
Fruit cocktail, canned in juice	4	L	M
Fruit cocktail, canned in syrup	4	M	L
Fruit salad, mixed	5	L	L
Golden raisins	0.6	M	H
Goji berries	0.3	L	L
Gooseberries	3.5	L	L
Gooseberries, canned in syrup	5	M	M
Gooseberries, stewed with sugar	5	M	M
Gooseberries, stewed without sugar	5	L	L
Grapefruit	8	L	L
Grapefruit, canned in juice	4.2	L	L
Grapefruit, canned in syrup	4.2	L	M
Grapes, green	3.5	L	L
Grapes, red	3.5	L	L
Greengages	3.5	L	L
Greengages, stewed with sugar	3.5	M	M
Greengages, stewed without sugar	3.5	L	L
Guavas	3.5	L	L
Guavas, canned in syrup	4	M	M
Kiwi fruit	2	L	L
Kumquats	0.3	L	L
Kumquats, canned in syrup	0.3	M	M
Lemons, unpeeled	2	L	L
Limes, unpeeled	1.4	L	L
Loganberries, canned in juice	5	L	L
Loganberries, stewed with sugar	5	M	M
Loganberries, stewed without sugar	5	L	L
Lychees	3.2	L	L
Lychees, canned in syrup	2.8	M	H

Unless otherwise stated, fruits are prepared but uncooked.

ENERGY cal	ENERGY J	FAT g	SATURATED FAT g	PROTEIN g	CARBO-HYDRATE g	FIBER g
124	530	Trace	Trace	2	31	1.8
162	691	1	0.1	2	41	2.4
109	460	1	Trace	2	23	3
24	102	1	0.1	1	5	0.8
176	747	1	Trace	3	41	5.8
33	140	Trace	Trace	0	8	1.2
66	281	Trace	Trace	0	17	1.2
77	332	Trace	Trace	1	19	2.1
50	211	Trace	Trace	0	12	0.4
33	138	0.2	0	1.4	6.9	0.5
40	170	1	0.1	1	9	2.4
102	434	Trace	Trace	1	26	2.4
76	321	Trace	Trace	1	18	2.7
22	92	Trace	Trace	1	4	2.8
291	Trace	Trace	2	16	3	
36	144	Trace	Trace	1	9	0.5
72	308	Trace	Trace	1	19	0.7
62	263	0.2	0	0.7	15.2	0.7
67	286	0.1	0	0.6	17	0.6
41	173	Trace	Trace	1	10	2.1
81	347	Trace	Trace	1	21	1.9
36	155	Trace	Trace	1	9	1.9
26	112	1	Trace	1	5	3.7
68	292	Trace	Trace	0	18	3.4
29	124	Trace	Trace	1	6	1.1
3	15	Trace	Trace	0	1	0.3
11	46	Trace	Trace	0	3	0.1
8	36	1	0.1	0	1	1.7
4	14	0	0	0	0	1.1
141	601	Trace	Trace	1	37	2.2
70	300	Trace	Trace	1	18	2.8
20	87	Trace	Trace	1	4	2.9
52	223	Trace	Trace	1	13	0.6
54	232	Trace	Trace	0	14	0.4

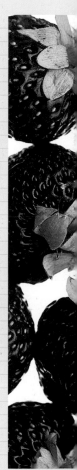

FRUITS	AVERAGE PORTION oz	GI	GL
Mandarin oranges, canned in juice	4	L	L
Mandarin oranges, canned in syrup	4.4	L	M
Mangoes	5.3	L	L
Mangoes, canned in syrup	3.7	M	L
Mangosteen	2	L	L
Melon, Canteloupe	5.3	H	H
Melon, Galia	5.3	H	H
Melon, Honeydew	7	H	H
Mixed candied peel	0.2	H	H
Nectarines	5.3	L	L
Oranges	5.6	L	L
Passion fruit	2	L	L
Paw-paw	5	M	L
Peaches	3.9	L	L
Peaches, canned in juice	4.2	L	L
Peaches, canned in syrup	4.2	M	M
Pears, canned in juice	4.7	L	L
Pears, canned in syrup	4.7	M	M
Pears, Comice	5.3	L	L
Pears, Conference	6	M	M
Pears, Nashi	5.3	L	L
Pears, William	5.3	L	L
Pineapple	2.8	M	L
Pineapple, canned in juice	1.4	L	L
Pineapple, canned in syrup	1.4	M	M
Plums, average, stewed with sugar	4.7	M	M
Plums, average, stewed without sugar	2.5	L	L
Plums, canned in syrup	2.8	M	M
Plums, Victoria	1.9	L	L
Plums, yellow	1.9	L	L
Pomegranate	1.9	L	L
Pomelo	2.8	L	L
Prickly pears	2.8	L	L
Prunes, canned in juice	0.8	L	L

Unless otherwise stated, fruits are prepared but uncooked.

ENERGY cal	ENERGY J	FAT g	SATURATED FAT g	PROTEIN g	CARBO-HYDRATE g	FIBER g
37	155	Trace	Trace	1	9	0.3
66	281	Trace	Trace	1	17	0.3
86	368	1	0.2	1	21	3.9
81	347	Trace	Trace	0	21	0.7
44	184	Trace	Trace	0	10	1
29	122	Trace	Trace	1	6	1.5
36	153	Trace	Trace	1	8	0.6
56	238	Trace	Trace	1	13	1.2
12	49	Trace	Trace	0	3	0.2
60	257	Trace	Trace	2	14	1.8
58	243	0.3	0	1.3	13.1	2.7
22	91	1	0.1	2	3	2
50	214	Trace	Trace	1	12	3.1
36	156	Trace	Trace	1	8	1.7
47	198	Trace	Trace	1	12	1
66	280	Trace	Trace	1	17	1.1
45	190	Trace	Trace	0	11	1.9
68	290	Trace	Trace	0	18	1.5
50	212	Trace	Trace	0	13	3
90	386	1	Trace	1	22	4.1
44	183	Trace	Trace	0	11	2.3
51	215	Trace	Trace	1	12	3.3
33	141	Trace	Trace	0	8	1
19	80	Trace	Trace	0	5	0.2
26	109	Trace	Trace	0	7	0.3
105	446	Trace	Trace	1	27	1.7
21	90	Trace	Trace	0	5	0.9
47	202	Trace	Trace	0	12	0.6
21	92	Trace	Trace	0	5	1
14	59	Trace	Trace	0	3	0.6
28	120	Trace	Trace	1	6	1.9
24	101	Trace	Trace	0	5	0.8
29	124	1	0.1	0	7	2.2
19	80	Trace	Trace	0	5	0.6

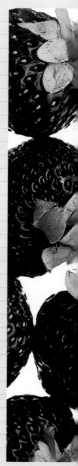

FRUITS	AVERAGE PORTION oz	GI	GL
Prunes, canned in syrup	0.8	L	L
Prunes, dried	2.3	M	L
Prunes, stewed with sugar	0.8	M	M
Prunes, stewed without sugar	0.8	L	L
Quinces	3.2	L	L
Raisins	1	M	H
Rambutan	2.8	L	L
Raspberries	2	L	L
Raspberries, canned in syrup	3.2	M	M
Raspberries, stewed with sugar	3.2	M	M
Raspberries, stewed without sugar	3.2	L	L
Redcurrants	0.1	L	L
Redcurrants, stewed with sugar	5	M	M
Redcurrants, stewed without sugar	5	L	L
Rhubarb, canned in syrup	5	L	L
Rhubarb, stewed with sugar	5	M	M
Rhubarb, stewed without sugar	5	L	L
Satsumas	2.5	L	L
Sharon fruit	3.9	M	L
Starfruit	4.2	L	L
Strawberries	3.5	L	L
Sugar apples	2	L	L
Tangerines	2.5	L	L
Watermelon	7	H	H

Unless otherwise stated, fruits are prepared but uncooked.

ENERGY cal	ENERGY J	FAT g	SATURATED FAT g	PROTEIN g	CARBO- HYDRATE g	FIBER g
22	93	Trace	Trace	0	6	0.7
93	397	Trace	Trace	2	22	3.8
25	105	Trace	Trace	0	6	0.7
19	83	Trace	0	0	5	0.8
23	99	Trace	Trace	0	6	1.7
82	348	Trace	Trace	1	21	0.6
55	234	Trace	Trace	1	13	0.5
15	65	1	0.1	1	3	1.5
79	337	Trace	Trace	1	20	1.4
57	244	1	0.1	1	14	2
22	95	1	0.1	1	4	2.2
0	2	Trace	Trace	0	0	0.1
74	318	Trace	Trace	1	19	3.8
24	106	Trace	Trace	1	5	4.1
43	182	Trace	Trace	1	11	1.1
67	284	Trace	Trace	1	16	1.7
10	42	Trace	Trace	1	1	1.8
25	109	Trace	Trace	1	6	0.9
80	342	Trace	Trace	1	20	1.8
38	163	1	0.1	1	9	1.6
30	126	0.5	0.1	0.6	6.1	1
41	178	Trace	Trace	1	10	1.4
25	103	Trace	Trace	1	6	0.9
62	266	1	0.2	1	14	0.2

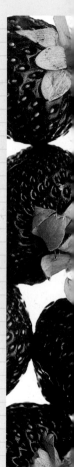

VEGETABLES	AVERAGE PORTION oz	GI	GL
Ackee, canned	2.8	L	L
Alfalfa sprouts	0.2	L	L
Artichoke, globe, heart	1.4	L	L
Artichoke, Jerusalem	2	M	L
Arugula leaves	0.7	L	L
Asparagus	4.4	L	L
Bamboo shoots, canned	1.8	L	L
Beans			
Aduki, dried, boiled	2	L	L
Baked, canned in tomato sauce	4.8	L	L
Baked, canned in tomato sauce, reduced sugar and salt	4.8	M	M
Balor, canned	4.8	L	L
Barbecue, canned in sauce	4.8	M	M
Blackeyed, dried, boiled	2	L	M
Broad	4.2	H	L
Broad, canned	4.2	H	L
Broad, frozen	4.2	H	L
Butter, canned	4.2	L	L
Butter, dried, boiled	2	L	L
Chili, canned	4.8	L	L
Edamame (soybean)	0.8	L	L
French	3.2	L	L
French, canned	3.2	L	L
French, frozen	3.2	L	L
Garbanzo (chickpea), canned	2.5	L	L
Garbanzo (chickpea), split, dried, boiled	2.5	L	L
Garbanzo (chickpea), whole, dried, boiled	2.5	L	L
Green, boiled	3.2	L	L
Green, canned	3.2	L	L
Green, frozen	3.2	L	L
Green, raw	3.2	L	L

Unless otherwise stated, vegetables are described as they would normally be eaten.

ENERGY cal	ENERGY J	FAT g	SATURATED FAT g	PROTEIN g	CARBO- HYDRATE g	FIBER g
121	500	12	Trace	2	1	1.4
1	5	Trace	Trace	0	0	0.1
7	31	0	0	1	1	2
23	116	Trace	Trace	1	6	2
4	15	0.1	0	0.7	0	0.3
33	138	1	0.1	4	2	1.7
6	23	1	0.1	1	0	0.9
74	315	Trace	Trace	6	14	3.3
109	463	0.7	0.1	6.8	20.3	5.1
99	420	1	0.1	7	17	5.1
26	112	Trace	Trace	3	4	3.6
104	444	1	0.1	7	19	4.7
70	296	1	0.1	5	12	2.1
58	245	1	0.1	6	7	6.5
104	444	1	0.1	10	15	6.2
97	413	1	0.1	9	14	7.8
92	392	1	0.1	7	16	5.5
62	262	1	0.1	4	11	3.1
95	513	1	0.1	7	16	5.3
111	464	5.2	0.8	10	4	3.7
20	83	1	0.1	2	3	2.2
20	86	Trace	Trace	1	4	2.3
23	97	Trace	Trace	2	4	3.7
81	341	2	0.2	5	11	2.9
80	339	1	0.1	5	12	3
85	358	1	0.1	6	13	3
23	98	0.3	1.8	1.9	3.6	2.3
20	86	Trace	Trace	1	4	2.3
23	97	Trace	Trace	2	4	3.7
21	89	0.4	2.9	1.9	2.8	2.3

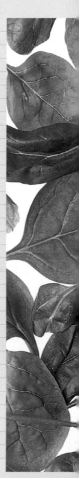

VEGETABLES	AVERAGE PORTION oz	GI	GL
Lilva, canned	2.8	L	L
Mung, dahl, dried, boiled	2	L	L
Mung, whole, dried, boiled	2	L	L
Navy, dried, boiled	2	L	M
Papri, canned	2	L	L
Pigeon peas, dahl, dried	2	L	L
Pinto, dried, boiled	2	L	L
Pinto, refried	2	L	L
Red kidney, canned	2	L	L
Red kidney, dried, boiled	2	L	L
Runner	3.2	L	L
Soy, dried, boiled	2	L	L
Beansprouts, mung	2.8	L	L
Beansprouts, mung, canned	2.8	L	L
Beansprouts, mung, stir-fried	2.8	L	L
Beet (beetroot)	1.4	M	L
Beet (beetroot), pickled	1.2	M	L
Belgian endive, raw	1	L	L
Bell peppers, green	5.6	L	L
Bell peppers, red	3.5	L	L
Bell peppers, red, cooked	3.5	L	L
Bell peppers, yellow	5.6	L	L
Bok choy, steamed	3.2	L	L
Breadfruit, canned	1.4	L	L
Broccoli, green	3	L	L
Broccoli, purple sprouting	3	L	L
Brussels sprouts	3.2	L	L
Cabbage, green	3.4	L	L
Cabbage, green, raw	3.2	L	L
Cabbage, Napa	1.4	L	L
Cabbage, red	3.2	L	L
Cabbage, red, raw	3.2	L	L
Cabbage, Savoy	3.4	L	L
Cabbage, white	3.4	L	L

Unless otherwise stated, vegetables are described as they would normally be eaten.

ENERGY cal	ENERGY J	FAT g	SATURATED FAT g	PROTEIN g	CARBO- HYDRATE g	FIBER g
54	232	1	0.1	5	8	0.5
55	235	1	0.1	5	9	1.8
55	233	1	0.1	5	9	1.8
57	244	1	0.1	4	10	3.7
16	66	1	0.1	2	2	0.4
71	298	1	0.1	5	13	4
82	350	1	0.1	5	14	2.8
64	268	1	0.1	4	9	3.2
60	254	1	0.1	4	11	3.7
62	264	1	0.1	5	10	4
16	68	1	0.1	1	2	1.7
85	354	4	0.5	8	3	3.7
25	105	1	0.1	2	3	1.2
8	35	Trace	Trace	1	1	0.6
58	238	5	0.4	2	2	0.7
18	78	Trace	Trace	1	4	0.8
10	41	Trace	Trace	0	2	0.6
3	13	1	0.1	0	1	0.3
24	104	1	0.2	1	4	2.6
29	121	0.2	0.1	0.8	6.4	1
46	193	0.1	0	0.8	11.2	0.8
42	181	Trace	Trace	2	8	2.7
13	53	0.1	1.8	1.4	1.7	0.9
26	112	Trace	Trace	0	7	0.7
20	85	1	0.2	3	1	2
16	68	1	0.1	2	1	2
32	138	1	0.3	3	3	2.8
24	103	0.2	0	2.2	3.7	2.4
16	67	0.2	0	1.4	2.2	2.5
5	20	Trace	Trace	0	1	0.5
14	55	Trace	Trace	1	2	1.8
19	80	Trace	Trace	1	3	2.3
16	67	1	0.1	1	2	1.9
13	57	Trace	Trace	1	2	1.4

VEGETABLES	AVERAGE PORTION oz	GI	GL
Cabbage, white, raw	3.2	L	L
Carrots, canned	2	M	L
Carrots, old, boiled	2	M	L
Carrots, old, raw	2.8	M	L
Carrots, young	2	M	L
Carrots, young, raw	2	M	L
Cassava, baked	3.5	M	M
Cauliflower, boiled	3.2	L	L
Cauliflower, raw	3.2	L	L
Celeriac (celery root)	1	L	L
Celeriac, raw	1	L	L
Celery	1	L	L
Chard, Swiss	3.2	L	L
Chili peppers, capsicum red	0.3	L	L
Chinese leaf	1.4	L	L
Corn, baby, canned	2	M	M
Corn kernels, boiled on cob	3	M	M
Corn kernels, canned	3	M	M
Cucumber	0.8	L	L
Curly endive	1	L	L
Curly kale	3.4	L	L
Curly kale, boiled	3.5	L	L
Eggplant, fried	4.6	L	L
Fennel	1.4	L	L
Garlic, raw	0.1	L	L
Jackfruit, canned	2	L	L
Kohlrabi	2	L	L
Kohlrabi, cooked	3.2	L	L
Leeks	2.6	L	L
Lentils, canned in tomato sauce	2.8	M	L
Lentils, green or brown, whole, dried	2.8	L	L
Lentils, red, split, dried, boiled	2.8	L	L
Lettuce	2.8	L	L
Mixed vegetables, frozen	3.2	L	L

Unless otherwise stated, vegetables are described as they would normally be eaten.

ENERGY cal	ENERGY J	FAT g	SATURATED FAT g	PROTEIN g	CARBO-HYDRATE g	FIBER g
22	91	0.1	0	1.1	4.3	1.8
12	52	1	0.1	0	3	1.1
66	275	0.3	0	0.3	2.9	1.3
27	117	0.3	0.1	0.4	6.2	1.7
13	56	1	0.1	0	3	1.4
18	75	1	0.1	0	4	1.4
155	661	1	0.1	1	40	1.7
21	89	0.8	0.2	1.7	1.9	1.4
27	108	0.4	0	2.3	4	1.6
5	19	Trace	Trace	0	1	1
5	22	Trace	Trace	0	1	1.1
2	10	Trace	Trace	0	0	0.3
18	76	Trace	Trace	2	3	1.8
3	11	Trace	Trace	0	0	0.1
5	20	Trace	Trace	0	1	0.5
14	58	Trace	Trace	2	1	0.9
57	241	1.6	0.2	3.1	8.1	2.2
107	446		1.4	0.2	2.2	22.6
3	15	0.2	0	0.3	0.3	0.2
4	16	0	0	1	0	0.6
23	95	1	0.2	2	1	2.7
24	100	1.1	0.2	2.4	1	2.8
393	1620	41	5.3	2	4	3
5	20	Trace	Trace	0	1	1
3	12	0	0	0	0	0.1
62	264	Trace	Trace	0	16	0.9
14	57	Trace	Trace	1	2	1.3
16	69	Trace	Trace	1	3	1.7
16	65	1	0.1	1	2	1.3
44	189	Trace	Trace	4	7	1.4
84	357	1	0.1	7	14	3
80	339	Trace	Trace	6	14	1.5
12	49	0.4	0.1	1	1.1	1
38	162	Trace	Trace	3	6	2.9

VEGETABLES	AVERAGE PORTION oz	GI	GL
Mushrooms			
Shiitake, steamed	1.4	L	L
Straw, canned	1.4	L	L
White, cooked in sunflower oil	1.5	L	L
White, raw	1.4	L	L
White, stewed	1.4	L	L
Okra	1	L	L
Onions, raw	5.3	L	L
Onions, fried	1.4	L	L
Parsley, fresh	0.3	L	L
Parsnips	2.3	H	M
Parsnips, roasted without oil	3.2	H	M
Peas, canned	2.5	M	L
Peas, fresh	2.5	M	L
Peas, frozen	2.5	L	L
Peas, frozen, microwaved	2.5	L	L
Peas, marrowfat, canned	2.8	M	L
Peas, petit pois, canned	2.5	M	L
Peas, petit pois, frozen	2.5	M	L
Peas, sugar-snap	3.2	L	L
Plantain	7	L	M
Plantain, ripe, fried	7	L	M
Potatoes and potato products			
Duchesse	4.2	H	H
Fries, crinkle cut, frozen, fried	5.8	H	H
Fries, French	5.8	H	H
Fries, frozen, baked	5.8	H	H
Fries, microwave	5.8	H	H
Fries, shoestring, frozen, fried	5.8	H	H
Fries, straight cut, frozen, fried	5.8	H	H
Instant, made with low-fat milk	2	H	M
Instant, made with water	2	H	M
Instant, made with whole milk	2	H	M
New, canned	5.8	M	M

Unless otherwise stated, vegetables are described as they would normally be eaten.

ENERGY cal	ENERGY J	FAT g	SATURATED FAT g	PROTEIN g	CARBO-HYDRATE g	FIBER g
22	93	Trace	0	1	5	0.8
6	25	Trace	Trace	1	0	1
48	202	4.8	0.9	1.1	0.1	0.7
3	12	0.1	0	0.4	0.1	0.5
4	15	0.1	0	0.6	0	0.8
8	36	1	0.1	1	1	1.1
53	225	0.2	0	1.5	12	1.7
66	274	4	0.6	1	6	1.2
3	14	0.1	0	0.3	0.3	0.5
43	181	1	0.1	1	8	3.1
102	427	6	Trace	1	12	4.2
56	237	1	0.1	4	9	3.6
55	230	1	0.2	5	7	3.2
48	202	0.5	0.1	3.7	7.5	2.7
50	212	0.6	0.1	4	7.6	3.2
80	329	1	0.1	6	14	3.3
32	132	1	0.1	4	3	3
34	144	1	0.1	4	4	3.2
30	125	1	0.1	3	4	1.2
224	954	1	0.2	2	57	2.4
534	2252	1	2	3	95	4.6
148	622	6	3.6	4	20	1.4
479	2001	28	5.1	6	55	3.6
312	1313	11	1.5	6	50	3.6
267	1134	7	3	5	49	3.3
365	1535	17	3	6	53	4.8
601	2515	35	6.6	7	68	4.5
450	1889	22	4.1	7	59	4
42	178	1	0.2	1	9	0.6
34	147	Trace	Trace	1	8	0.6
46	193	1	0.4	1	9	0.6
104	447	Trace	Trace	2	25	1.3

VEGETABLES	AVERAGE PORTION oz	GI	GL
New, fried	5.8	H	H
New, in skins, boiled	6.2	H	M
Old, baked	6.3	H	M
Old, boiled	6.2	H	M
Old, mashed with butter	4.2	H	M
Old, mashed with polyunsaturated fat spread	4.2	H	M
Old, microwaved	6.3	H	M
Old, roasted	4.6	H	M
Shaped potato products, baked	3.5	H	H
Steak fries, frozen, baked	5.8	H	H
Steak fries, frozen, fried	5.8	H	H
Waffles, frozen	3.2	H	H
Wedges, baked	6.3	H	H
Pumpkin	2	H	L
Radicchio, raw	1	L	L
Radishes, red, raw	1.7	L	L
Rosemary, fresh	0.3	L	L
Rutabaga	2	H	L
Salad onions	0.3	L	L
Sauerkraut	1	L	L
Scallions	0.3	L	L
Shallots	3.5	L	L
Snow peas, stir-fried	3.2	L	L
Spinach	3.2	L	L
Spinach, baby	3.2	L	L
Spinach, cooked	3.2	L	L
Split peas, dried, boiled	3.2	L	L
Spring greens, boiled	3.4	L	L
Squash, acorn, baked	2.3	L	L
Squash, butternut, baked	2.3	L	L
Squash, spaghetti, baked	2.3	L	L
Sweet potato	4.6	L	M
Sweet potato, baked	4.6	M	H

Unless otherwise stated, vegetables are described as they would normally be eaten.

ENERGY cal	ENERGY J	FAT g	SATURATED FAT g	PROTEIN g	CARBO-HYDRATE g	FIBER g
376	1582	16	2	7	55	2.8
119	509	1.1	0.2	3.2	26.1	1.6
175	743	0.4	0	4.5	40.7	2.5
130	551	0.2	0	3.2	30.6	1.8
125	526	5	3.4	2	19	1.3
125	526	5	1.1	2	19	1.3
166	706	0.2	0	4.7	38.7	2.5
194	819	6	0.8	4	34	2.3
190	799	8.3	0.9	2.5	28.1	2.8
259	1096	67	2.8	5	46	3
386	1622	17	3.1	6	56	4
180	758	12	1	2	28	2
245	1046	Trace	Trace	7	57	4.9
8	34	1	0.1	0	1	0.7
4	17	Trace	Trace	0	1	0.5
6	24	0	0	0	1	0.4
10	42	0.4	0	0.4	1.4	0.5
7	28	Trace	Trace	0	1	0.4
2	10	0	0	0	0	0.2
3	11	Trace	Trace	0	0	0.7
2	10	0	0	0	0	0.2
21	88	0.4	0	1.4	3.2	1.4
64	268	4	0.4	3	3	2.2
23	93	1	0.1	3	1	1.9
11	45	0.1	0	2.3	0.2	1.1
17	71	1	0.1	2	1	1.9
113	484	1	0.2	7	20	2.4
19	78	1	0.1	2	2	2.5
36	152	Trace	Trace	1	8	2.1
21	89	Trace	Trace	1	5	0.9
15	62	Trace	0.1	0	3	1.4
109	465	1	0.1	1	27	3
150	634	1	0.3	2	36	4.3

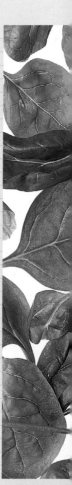

VEGETABLES	AVERAGE PORTION oz	GI	GL
Tarragon, fresh	0.3	L	L
Tomatoes, canned	7	L	L
Tomatoes, cherry	3.2	L	L
Tomatoes, fried	3	L	L
Tomatoes, grilled/broiled	3	L	L
Tomatoes, raw	3	L	L
Turnips	2	L	L
Water chestnuts, canned	1	L	L
Watercress	0.7	L	L
Yam	4.6	L	M
Yam, baked	4.6	M	M
Yam, steamed	4.6	M	M
Zucchini	3.2	L	L
Zucchini, fried	3.2	L	L

PREPARED SALADS			
Arugula salad	1	L	L
Baby leaf salad	1.8	L	L
Bean salad	7	L	L
Beet salad	3.5	M	L
Caesar salad with chicken, no dressing	7.6	L	L
Caesar salad with shrimps, no dressing	8.2	L	L
Carrot and nut salad with French dressing	3.4	L	L
Coleslaw, economy, store bought	3.5	L	L
Coleslaw, store bought	3.5	L	L
Coleslaw, with mayonnaise	3.5	L	L
Coleslaw, with reduced-calorie dressing	3.5	L	L
Coleslaw, with vinaigrette	3.5	L	L
Greek salad	3.4	L	L

Unless otherwise stated, vegetables are described as they would normally be eaten.

ENERGY cal	ENERGY J	FAT g	SATURATED FAT g	PROTEIN g	CARBO- HYDRATE g	FIBER g
5	21	0.1	0	0.3	0.6	0.5
38	160	0.2	0	2.2	7.6	1.4
18	74	0.2	0	1	3.2	1.1
77	320	7	0.9	1	4	1.1
14	57	0.1	0	0.5	2.9	0.9
14	57	0.3	0.1	0.4	2.6	0.9
7	31	1	Trace	0	1	1.1
9	37	Trace	Trace	0	3	2
4	19	1	0.1	1	0	0.3
173	738	1	0.1	2	43	1.8
199	846	1	0.1	3	49	2.2
148	634	1	0.1	2	37	1.7
17	73	1	0.1	2	2	1.1
57	239	4	0.5	2	2	1.1
3	12	Trace	Trace	Trace	Trace	0.2
9	40	Trace	Trace	Trace	2	0.7
294	1236	19	2	8	26	6
100	417	7	0.7	2	8	1.7
105	438	2	0.6	17	4	1
106	444	2	0.7	15	7	1
207	858	17	1.6	2	13	2.3
110	456	9.1	0.7	0.9	6.5	1.8
173	714	16.3	1.7	0.8	6	1.7
258	939	26	3.9	1	4	1.4
67	280	5	0.5	1	6	1.4
87	364	4	0.5	1	12	1.7
124	513	12	3.1	3	2	0.8

PREPARED SALADS

	AVERAGE PORTION oz	GI	GL
Green salad	3.4	L	L
Herb salad	1.8	L	L
Pasta salad	3.4	L	M
Pasta salad, whole-wheat	3.4	L	M
Potato salad, with mayonnaise	3	H	H
Potato salad, with reduced-calorie mayonnaise	3	H	H
Rice salad	3.2	H	H
Rice salad, brown	3.4	M	H
Taco salad	6.9	M	M
Tabbouleh	3.5	M	H
Tomato and onion salad	3.2	L	L
Vegetable salad, with shrimps, no dressing	8.2	L	L
Waldorf salad	3.2	L	L

VEGETABLE DISHES, HOMEMADE

	AVERAGE PORTION oz	GI	GL
Bhaji, pea, potato, and cauliflower	2.5	M	H
Bhaji, potato and cauliflower, fried	2.5	M	H
Bhaji, potato and onion	2.5	M	H
Broccoli in cheese sauce, made with low-fat milk	6.7	L	M
Broccoli in cheese sauce, made with whole milk	6.7	L	L
Cannelloni, spinach	12	M	H
Cannelloni, vegetable	12	M	H
Casserole, vegetable	7.8	M	H
Cauliflower in cheese sauce, made with low-fat milk	7	L	M
Cauliflower in cheese sauce, made with whole milk	7	L	M

Unless otherwise stated, vegetables are described as they would normally be eaten.

ENERGY cal	ENERGY J	FAT g	SATURATED FAT g	PROTEIN g	CARBO- HYDRATE g	FIBER g
11	48	0	Trace	1	2	1
9	40	Trace	Trace	Trace	Trace	0.7
121	473	7	1	2	13	1.5
124	493	7	1	3	13	2.6
203	757	18	2.6	1	10	0.8
82	349	3	0.3	1	13	0.7
149	628	7	1	3	21	0.6
159	668	7	1	3	23	1
279	1168	15	6.8	13	24	n/a
119	496	5	0.4	3	17	1
65	272	5	0.6	1	4	0.9
106	444	2	0.7	15	7	1
174	662	16	2.1	1	7	1.2
49	209	2	0.2	2	7	2
214	888	15	1.8	5	14	2.7
112	468	7	4.6	1	12	1.1
211	880	14	7.2	12	9	2.9
224	939	16	8.2	12	9	2.9
449	1880	26	7.8	15	43	2.7
493	2067	31	11.6	15	43	2.4
114	486	1	0.2	5	23	4.6
200	840	13	6	12	10	2.6
210	880	14	6.6	12	10	2.6

VEGETABLE DISHES, HOMEMADE	AVERAGE PORTION oz	GI	GL
Cauliflower in white sauce, made with low-fat milk	7	L	M
Cauliflower in white sauce, made with whole milk	7	L	M
Chili, bean and lentil	10	L	M
Chili, vegetable	7.9	L	L
Curry, chickpea	7.4	L	L
Curry, potato and pea	10	M	H
Curry, vegetable	7	L	L
Dahl, mung bean, dried, boiled	2	L	L
Dahl, pigeon peas, dried, boiled	2	L	L
Falafel, fried	3.5	L	M
Kiev, vegetable	5.3	M	M
Lasagne, spinach	15	M	H
Lasagne, spinach, whole-wheat	15	M	H
Lasagne, vegetarian	11.3	M	H
Moussaka, vegetable	14	L	M
Nut and vegetable roast	3.5	L	L
Pakora, potato and cauliflower, fried	2.5	M	M
Pâté, vegetable	3.5	L	L
Peppers, stuffed with rice	6.2	M	H
Peppers, stuffed with vegetables, cheese topping	6.2	M	M
Pilaf, mushroom	6.3	M	H
Pilaf, vegetable	6.3	M	H
Quiche, broccoli	5	H	H
Quiche, broccoli, whole-wheat	5	H	H
Quiche, cauliflower and cheese	5	H	H
Quiche, cauliflower and cheese, wholewheat	5	H	H
Quiche, cheese and egg	5	H	H
Quiche, cheese and egg, whole-wheat	5	H	H
Quiche, cheese and mushroom	5	H	H

Unless otherwise stated, vegetables are described as they would normally be eaten.

ENERGY cal	ENERGY J	FAT g	SATURATED FAT g	PROTEIN g	CARBO- HYDRATE g	FIBER g
122	512	6	2.2	7	10	2.2
136	568	8	3.2	7	10	2.2
264	1111	8	0.9	15	38	10.4
125	532	1	0.2	7	24	5.7
227	956	8	0.8	13	30	6.9
267	1122	11	1.2	8	38	7
176	736	12	1.2	5	14	5
55	235	1	0.1	5	9	1.8
71	298	1	0.1	5	13	4
179	750	11	1.1	6	16	3.4
280	1172	16.6	6.2	6.5	26.7	5.7
365	1541	13	5.5	15	53	4.6
391	1659	13	5.5	18	55	9.7
458	1930	19.5	9	23.7	50.2	2.2
280	1172	10.8	5.2	10.8	36.4	9.6
314	1311	21.9	3.2	11.1	19.6	3.9
214	888	15	1.8	5	14	2.7
173	718	13.4	4.6	7.5	5.9	1.5
149	630	4	0.7	3	27	2.3
194	810	12	3.5	6	17	2.6
248	1048	8	4.5	4	43	0.7
248	1053	8	4.3	5	43	1
349	1455	21	8.3	12	30	1.7
337	1408	21	8.3	13	25	3.8
277	1156	18	7.1	7	24	1.5
269	1121	18	7.1	8	20	3.1
440	1834	31	14.4	18	24	0.8
431	1796	31	14.6	18	20	2.7
396	1655	26	10.8	15	26	1.3

VEGETABLE DISHES, HOMEMADE	AVERAGE PORTION oz	GI	GL
Quiche, cheese and mushroom, wholewheat	5	H	H
Quiche, cheese, onion and potato	5	H	H
Quiche, cheese, onion and potato, wholewheat	5	H	H
Quiche, mushroom	5	H	H
Quiche, mushroom, whole-wheat	5	H	H
Quiche, spinach	5	H	H
Quiche, spinach, whole-wheat	5	H	H
Quiche, vegetable	5	H	H
Quiche, vegetable, whole-wheat	5	H	H
Refried beans	3.2	L	L
Rice and blackeye beans	7	M	M
Rice and blackeye beans, brown rice	7	M	M
Risotto, vegetable	10	M	H
Risotto, vegetable, brown rice	10	M	H
Vegetable bake	11.3	L	M
Vine leaves, stuffed with rice	2.8	L	M

VEGETARIAN PRODUCTS AND DISHES			
Beanburger	3.5	M	M
Hormel vegetarian chili with beans, canned	8.7	L	L
Quorn™, myco-protein	3.2	L	L
Quorn™ burger	1.8	L	L
Quorn™ grounds	3.5	L	L
Quorn™ nuggets	3.5	L	L
Quorn™ roast	3.5	L	L
Quorn™ sausage	1.8	L	L
Soy burger	3.5	L	L
Soy grounds	3.5	L	L
Tempeh	2	L	L

Unless otherwise stated, vegetables are described as they would normally be eaten.

ENERGY cal	ENERGY J	FAT g	SATURATED FAT g	PROTEIN g	CARBO-HYDRATE g	FIBER g
388	1616	27	10.8	16	22	3.1
480	2005	33	16	18	28	1.4
472	1966	34	16.1	19	25	3.1
398	1659	27	12.2	14	26	1.3
388	1618	28	12.2	15	21	3.1
287	1203	18	5.6	14	18	2
281	1176	18	5.6	15	16	3.2
295	1238	18	6	7	28	2.1
286	1197	18	6	8	24	3.9
211	885	12	2.7	9	18	6.3
366	1556	7	3	12	68	2.8
350	1488	7	3	11	66	3.6
426	1798	19	2.9	12	56	6.4
415	1749	19	2.6	12	54	7
419	1754	23	9.3	13.8	41.9	3
210	875	14	2.1	2	19	1
190	795	7.6	0.6	9.6	20.7	4.6
205	857	1	0.1	12	38	9.9
77	326	3	Trace	11	2	4.3
80	321	3.7	1.3	7.1	4.1	1.2
94	397	2	0.5	14.5	4.5	5.5
182	761	10.5	1.5	12	9.9	4
106	445	2	0.5	15	4.5	4.9
86	362	3.5	0.3	6.8	6	1.8
179	749	6	0.7	17.9	13.4	4.6
303	1270	18.7	1.5	29.1	5	1.7
116	485	6.5	1.3	11.1	5.6	2.6

VEGETARIAN PRODUCTS AND DISHES	AVERAGE PORTION oz	GI	GL
Tofu, fried	2.8	L	L
Tofu, steamed	2.8	L	L
Tofu, steamed, fried	2.8	L	L
Tofu burger, baked	0.3	M	M
Vegeburger, fried	2	M	M
Vegeburger, grilled	2	M	M

Unless otherwise stated, vegetables are described as they would normally be eaten.

ENERGY cal	ENERGY J	FAT g	SATURATED FAT g	PROTEIN g	CARBO- HYDRATE g	FIBER g
242	1011	20	2.3	17	3	1
58	243	3	0.4	6	1	1
209	869	14	2.3	19	2	1
11	45	0	0.1	1	1	0.2
137	571	10	1.7	9	4	2
110	460	6	1.7	9	4	2.4

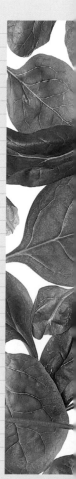

BEEF	AVERAGE PORTION oz	GI	GL
Flank, choice, braised	3	L	L
Flank, choice, broiled	3	L	L
Flank, choice, lean and fat, braised	3	L	L
Flank, choice, lean and fat, broiled	3	L	L
Flank, pot roasted	5	L	L
Flank, untrimmed, pot roasted	5	L	L
Ground, extra lean, stewed	5	L	L
Ground, medium, extra lean, baked	3	L	L
Ground, medium, extra lean, broiled	3	L	L
Ground, medium, extra lean, pan-fried	3	L	L
Ground, medium, lean, baked	3	L	L
Ground, medium, lean, broiled	3	L	L
Ground, medium, lean, pan-fried	3	L	L
Ground, medium, regular, baked	3	L	L
Ground, medium, regular, broiled	3	L	L
Ground, medium, regular, pan-fried	3	L	L
Meatballs, cooked	3.5	L	L
Rib eye steak, broiled	3.5	L	L
Rib, large end, choice, braised	3	L	L
Rib, large end, choice, lean and fat, braised	3	L	L
Rib, large end, choice, lean and fat, ¼" fat, braised	3	L	L
Rib, large end, choice, ¼" fat, braised	3	L	L
Rib, large end, prime, lean and fat, ½" fat, braised	3	L	L
Rib, large end, prime, lean and fat, ¼" fat, braised	3	L	L
Rib, large end, prime, ½" fat, braised	3	L	L
Rib, large end, prime, ¼" fat, braised	3	L	L
Rib, large end, select, braised	3	L	L
Rib, large end, select, lean and fat, braised	3	L	L

Unless otherwise stated, all meat is lean and trimmed, and all chops and cutlets are boned. Steaks are medium-sized. Unless otherwise stated, all dishes are homemade.

ENERGY cal	ENERGY J	FAT g	SATURATED FAT g	PROTEIN g	CARBO-HYDRATE g	FIBER g
201	843	11	4.7	24	0	0
176	736	9	3.7	23	0	0
224	935	14	5.9	23	0	0
192	804	11	4.5	22	0	0
354	1483	20	8	45	0	0
433	1800	31	12.7	38	0	0
248	1039	12	5.3	35	0	0
212	889	14	5.4	21	0	0
218	910	14	5.5	22	0	0
217	907	14	5.5	21	0	0
228	953	16	6.1	20	0	0
231	967	16	6.2	21	0	0
234	978	16	6.4	21	0	0
244	1021	18	7	20	0	0
246	1028	18	6.9	20	0	0
260	1088	19	7.5	20	0	0
195	814	13.2	5	12.4	7.6	0.5
155	649	8.3	3.2	20.1	0	0
215	900	13	5.1	23	0	0
316	1323	26	10.4	19	0	0
293	1227	26	10.8	13	0	0
204	853	12	5.1	21	0	0
326	1362	30	13	13	0	0
320	1340	29	12.3	13	0	0
250	1046	18	7.6	21	0	0
250	1046	18	7.6	21	0	0
187	782	10	3.9	23	0	0
281	1177	22	8.8	20	0	0

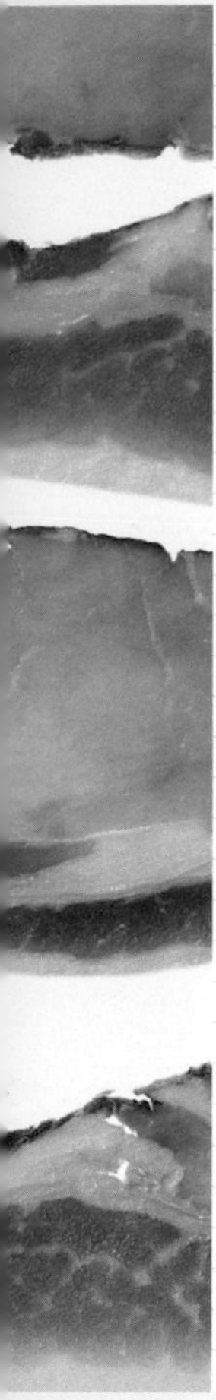

BEEF	AVERAGE PORTION oz	GI	GL
Rib, large end, select, lean and fat, ¼" fat, braised	3	L	L
Rib, large end, select, ¼" fat, braised	3	L	L
Rib, short, choice, braised	3	L	L
Rib, short, choice, lean and fat, braised	3	L	L
Rib, small end, choice, lean and fat, ¼" fat, braised	3	L	L
Rib, small end, choice, ¼" fat, braised	3	L	L
Rib, small end, prime, lean and fat, ½" fat, braised	3	L	L
Rib, small end, prime, lean and fat, ¼" fat, braised	3	L	L
Rib, small end, prime, ½" fat, braised	3	L	L
Rib, small end, prime, ¼" fat, braised	3	L	L
Rib roast, roasted	3.2	L	L
Rib roast, untrimmed, roasted	3.2	L	L
Short loin, porterhouse steak, choice, lean and fat, ¼" fat, broiled	8	L	L
Short loin, porterhouse steak, choice, ¼" fat, broiled	8	L	L
Short loin, porterhouse steak, select, lean and fat, ¼" fat, broiled	8	L	L
Short loin, porterhouse steak, select, ¼" fat, broiled	8	L	L
Short loin, t-bone steak, choice, lean and fat, ¼" fat, broiled	8	L	L
Short loin, t-bone steak, choice, ¼" fat, broiled	8	L	L
Short loin, t-bone steak, select, lean and fat, ¼" fat, broiled	8	L	L

Unless otherwise stated, all meat is lean and trimmed, and all chops and cutlets are boned. Steaks are medium-sized. Unless otherwise stated, all dishes are homemade.

ENERGY cal	ENERGY J	FAT g	SATURATED FAT g	PROTEIN g	CARBO- HYDRATE g	FIBER g
258	1081	22	9.1	14	0	0
175	733	9	3.8	21	0	0
251	1049	15	6.6	26	0	0
400	1675	36	15.1	18	0	0
268	1120	23	9.4	14	0	0
137	573	7	2.7	17	0	0
297	1241	26	11.3	14	0	0
291	1216	26	10.6	14	0	0
221	925	13	5.6	24	0	0
221	925	13	5.6	24	0	0
212	889	10	4.6	30	0	0
270	1125	18	8.3	26	0	0
580	2428	45	18	40	0	0
360	1505	18	6.7	46	0	0
500	2090	33	13.5	47	0	0
335	1402	13	4.9	51	0	0
536	2241	39	15.7	42	0	0
461	1930	23	8.1	60	0	0
443	1854	28	11.5	44	0	0

LAMB	AVERAGE PORTION oz	GI	GL
Leg, roasted medium	3.2	L	L
Leg, roasted well done	3.2	L	L
Leg, untrimmed, roasted medium	3.2	L	L
Leg, untrimmed, roasted well done	3.2	L	L
Leg chops, untrimmed, broiled	2.5	L	L
Leg half fillet, braised	2.5	L	L
Leg half fillet, untrimmed, braised	2.5	L	L
Leg half knuckle, pot roasted	3.2	L	L
Leg half knuckle, untrimmed, pot roasted	3.2	L	L
Leg roast, roasted	3.2	L	L
Leg roast, untrimmed, roasted	3.2	L	L
Leg steaks, broiled	3.2	L	L
Leg steaks, untrimmed, broiled	3.2	L	L
Loin chops, broiled	2.5	L	L
Loin chops, untrimmed, broiled	2.5	L	L
Loin chops, roasted	2.5	L	L
Loin chops, untrimmed, roasted	2.5	L	L
Loin roast, roasted	3.2	L	L
Loin roast, untrimmed, roasted	3.2	L	L
Shoulder half bladeside, pot roasted	3.2	L	L
Shoulder half bladeside, untrimmed, pot roasted	3.2	L	L
Shoulder half knuckle, braised	3.2	L	L
Shoulder half knuckle, untrimmed, braised	3.2	L	L
Shoulder joint, roasted	3.2	L	L
Shoulder joint, untrimmed, roasted	3.2	L	L
Shoulder, roasted	3.2	L	L
Shoulder, untrimmed, roasted	3.2	L	L

Unless otherwise stated, all meat is lean and trimmed, and all chops and cutlets are boned. Steaks are medium-sized. Unless otherwise stated, all dishes are homemade.

ENERGY cal	ENERGY J	FAT g	SATURATED FAT g	PROTEIN g	CARBO- HYDRATE g	FIBER g
183	768	8	3.4	27	0	0
187	786	8	3.3	28	0	0
216	904	13	5.3	25	0	0
218	909	12	5.1	27	0	0
155	648	8	3.5	20	0	0
143	597	7	3.2	19	0	0
179	748	12	5.4	18	0	0
181	760	8	3.5	26	0	0
213	889	12	5.4	25	0	0
189	791	9	3.1	28	0	0
212	887	12	4.2	27	0	0
178	746	8	3.2	26	0	0
208	868	12	5	25	0	0
149	624	7	3.4	20	0	0
214	888	15	7.4	19	0	0
180	754	9	4.3	24	0	0
251	1043	19	9	20	0	0
188	788	10	4.4	25	0	0
273	1133	20	9.5	23	0	0
211	878	13	5.8	24	0	0
292	1212	23	10.8	21	0	0
191	797	11	4.9	23	0	0
272	1130	21	9.7	21	0	0
212	884	12	5.6	26	0	0
254	1056	18	8.4	23	0	0
196	819	11	5	24	0	0
268	1114	20	9.4	22	0	0

MEAT DISHES AND PRODUCTS	AVERAGE PORTION oz	GI	GL
Beef bourguignon	9.2	M	M
Beef casserole, canned	9.5	H	**H**
Beef casserole, made with canned cook-in sauce	10.5	M	M
Beef pot pie, frozen	7	M	L
Beef sausages, broiled	1.4	M	M
Beef sausages, fried	1.4	M	M
Beef stew	9.8	M	M
Beef stew, made with lean beef	9.2	M	M
Beef stew and dumplings	9.2	H	H
Bologna, beef	1.6	M	L
Bologna, beef and pork	1.6	M	L
Bologna, pork	1.6	M	L
Bratwurst	2.6	M	L
Chili con carne	7.8	M	M
Chili con carne, canned	7.9	M	L
Chili con carne, store bought	7.8	M	M
Chili with beans, canned	9	M	L
Chorizo	1	L	L
Corned beef	1.8	M	L
Corned beef, brisket, cooked	3	M	L
Corned beef, canned	1.9	M	L
Corned beef hash	10.5	H	H
Corned beef loaf, jellied	1.9	M	L
Enchilada, with cheese	5.4	M	L
Enchilada, with cheese and beef	6.7	M	L
Hamburgers, broiled	3.5	M	L
Hamburgers, fried	3.5	M	L
Hamburgers, low-fat, broiled	3.5	M	L
Hamburgers, low-fat, fried	3.5	M	L
Hamburgers in gravy, canned	3.5	M	L
Hormel chili with beans, canned	8.7	M	L
Hormel chili, no beans, canned	8.3	M	L
Hormel, Wrangler beef franks	3.9	M	L

Unless otherwise stated, all meat is lean and trimmed, and all chops and cutlets are boned. Steaks are medium-sized. Unless otherwise stated, all dishes are homemade.

ENERGY cal	ENERGY J	FAT g	SATURATED FAT g	PROTEIN g	CARBO-HYDRATE g	FIBER g	
328	1368	17	5.5	36	7	1	
211	886	7	3.8	19	19	2.7	
408	1707	20	8.1	45	14	2.7	
449	1881	24	8.5	13	44	2.2	
111	463	8	3.2	5	5	0.3	
112	464	8	3	5	5	0.3	
316	1328	14	4.2	34	14	2	
263	1102	9	2.3	32	13	1.8	
499	2090	27	12.5	26	41	2.6	
144	600	13	5.6	6	0	0	
145	608	13	4.9	5	1	0	
114	475	9	3.2	7	0	0	
195	811	16	6	12	2	Trace	
286	1199	17	6.6	20	10	2.4	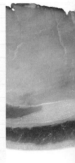
255	1068	8	2.1	20	24	8.2	
211	889	9	4.2	17	16	3.1	
287	1201	14	6	15	30	11.3	
87	362	7	2.9	5	1	Trace	
103	430	5	2.8	13	1	0	
213	892	16	5.4	15	0	0	
140	586	8	3.5	15	0	0	
423	1776	18	9.9	31	37	3	
87	365	3	1.5	13	0	0	
319	1337	19	10.6	10	29	n/a	
323	1350	18	9	12	30	n/a	
287	1194	20	8.8	25	1	0.2	
303	1261	23	8.7	24	1	0.2	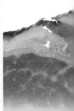
178	745	10	4.4	23	1	0	
193	807	11	5	24	0	0	
171	713	12	4.8	12	5	Trace	
240	1003	4	1.8	17	34	8.4	
194	809	7	2.2	17	18	3.1	
325	1360	29	11.9	14	2	0	

MEAT DISHES AND PRODUCTS	AVERAGE PORTION oz	GI	GL
Lebanon bologna, beef	46	M	L
Liver sausage/wurst, pork	1.2	M	L
Meatloaf	3.5	M	M
Mortadella	0.8	M	L
Moussaka	11.6	H	H
Moussaka, store bought	11.6	H	H
Nalley chili con carne, canned	9.1	M	L
Nestlé, Chef-Mate chili with beans, canned	8.9	M	L
Nestlé, Chef-Mate chili without beans, canned	8.8	M	L
Nestlé, Chef-Mate spicy chili with beans, canned	8.9	M	L
Old El Paso chili with beans, canned	7.9	M	L
Oscar Mayer wieners	1.6	M	L
Oscar Mayer wieners (bun length)	2	M	L
Oscar Mayer wieners, fat free	1.7	M	L
Oscar Mayer wieners, light	2	M	L
Pastrami	1	L	L
Pork and beef meatballs in tomato sauce	5.6	M	M
Pork and beef sausages, broiled	1.4	M	M
Pork, cured, ham, patties, broiled	2	M	M
Pork sausages, broiled	1.4	M	M
Pork sausages, fried	1.4	M	M
Pork sausages, frozen, broiled	1.4	M	M
Pork sausages, frozen, fried	1.4	M	M
Pork sausages, reduced-fat, broiled	1.4	M	M
Pork sausages, reduced-fat, fried	1.4	M	M
Premium sausages, broiled	1.4	M	M
Premium sausages, fried	1.4	M	M
Salami	1	L	L
Stagg classic chili with beans, canned	8.7	M	L
Stagg country chili with beans, canned	8.7	M	L

Unless otherwise stated, all meat is lean and trimmed, and all chops and cutlets are boned. Steaks are medium-sized. Unless otherwise stated, all dishes are homemade.

ENERGY cal	ENERGY J	FAT g	SATURATED FAT g	PROTEIN g	CARBO-HYDRATE g	FIBER g
98	408	6	2.7	9	1	0
117	491	10	3.8	5	1	0
214	894	11	4.1	17	13	0.5
79	328	7	2.8	3	0	Trace
403	1680	26	11.9	28	15	3.3
462	1934	27	9.6	27	28	2.6
281	1176	8	2.8	40	12	12.9
412	1725	25	10.9	18	29	11.1
430	1800	32	14.4	19	18	3
423	1768	25	10.7	17	33	4.3
249	1040	0	2.1	18	22	9.8
143	599	13	5.6	5	1	0
184	768	17	7.1	6	2	0
39	163	0	0.1	7	3	0
110	461	8	3.6	6	2	0
37	155	1.3	0.5	5.8	0.5	0
202	840	12	4.4	16	8	1.2
108	448	8	3	5	4	0.5
205	859	19	6.7	8	1	0
118	488	9	3.2	6	4	0.3
123	512	10	3.4	6	4	0.3
116	482	8	3	6	4	0.3
126	525	10	3.5	6	4	0.3
92	384	6	2	6	4	0.6
84	352	5	1.7	6	4	0.6
117	486	9	3.3	7	3	0.3
110	457	8	3.1	6	3	0.3
131	544	11.8	4.4	6.3	0.1	0
324	1354	16	6.7	17	29	7.4
319	1334	16	6.8	15	29	5.9

MEAT DISHES AND PRODUCTS	AVERAGE PORTION oz	GI	GL
Stagg Dynamite chili with beans, canned	8.7	M	M
Stagg Ranchhouse chili with beans, canned	8.7	M	M
Stagg Silverado chili with beans, canned	8.7	M	M
Vienna sausage, canned, beef and pork	4	L	L
Worthington Foods, Morningstar Farms deli franks	1.7	M	L
Worthington Foods, Morningstar Farms breakfast patties	1.7	M	L

VARIETY MEATS			
Heart, beef, stewed	7	L	L
Heart, lamb, roasted	7	L	L
Heart, lamb, stewed	7	L	L
Heart, pork, stewed	3.5	L	L
Kidney, beef, stewed	4	L	L
Kidney, lamb, fried	1.3	L	L
Kidney, pork, fried	5	L	L
Kidney, pork, stewed	5	L	L
Liver, beef, stewed	2.5	L	L
Liver, calf, fried	3.5	L	L
Liver, chicken, fried	2.5	L	L
Liver, lamb, fried	2.5	L	L
Liver, pork, stewed	2.5	L	L

PORK, BACON, AND HAM			
Bacon			
Hormel Canadian style bacon	2	L	L
Pork, cured, bacon, broiled, pan-fried or roasted	0.7	L	L
Pork, cured, Canadian-style bacon, grilled	1.7	L	L

Unless otherwise stated, all meat is lean and trimmed, and all chops and cutlets are boned. Steaks are medium-sized. Unless otherwise stated, all dishes are homemade.

ENERGY cal	ENERGY J	FAT g	SATURATED FAT g	PROTEIN g	CARBO-HYDRATE g	FIBER g
333	1396	15	5.7	18	31	8.2
284	1188	9	2.6	19	32	8.6
227	951	3	1	18	33	8.2
315	1319	28	10.5	12	2	0
112	467	6	0.9	10	4	2.7
79	332	3	0.5	10	4	2
314	1322	10	5	56	0	0
452	1888	28	6.2	51	0	0
312	1308	15	6	24	20	0
162	678	7	1.3	25	0	0
155	648	5	1.6	27	0	0
66	274	4	0.4	8	0	0
283	1187	13	2.1	41	0	0
214	897	9	2.8	34	0	0
139	582	7	2.5	17	2	0
176	734	10	2.7	22	Trace	0
118	494	6	3.5	15	Trace	0
237	989	13	4.9	30	Trace	0
132	555	6	1.8	18	2	0
68	286	3	1	9	1	0
109	458	9	3.3	6	0	0
87	364	4	1.3	11	1	0

PORK, BACON, AND HAM	AVERAGE PORTION oz	GI	GL
Blade chops, bone-in, braised	3	L	L
Blade chops, bone-in, broiled	3	L	L
Blade chops, bone-in, lean and fat, braised	3	L	L
Blade chops, bone-in, lean and fat, broiled	3	L	L
Blade chops, bone-in, lean and fat, pan-fried	3	L	L
Blade chops, bone-in, pan-fried	3	L	L
Blade roast, bone-in, lean and fat, roasted	3	L	L
Blade roast, bone-in, roasted	3	L	L
Boston blade roast, lean and fat, roasted	3	L	L
Boston blade roast, roasted	3	L	L
Boston blade steak, braised	3	L	L
Boston blade steak, broiled	3	L	L
Boston blade steak, lean and fat, braised	3	L	L
Boston blade steak, lean and fat, broiled	3	L	L
Center loin chops, bone-in, braised	3	L	L
Center loin chops, bone-in, broiled	3	L	L
Center loin chops, bone-in, lean and fat, braised	3	L	L
Center loin chops, bone-in, lean and fat, broiled	3	L	L
Center loin chops, bone-in, lean and fat, pan-fried	3	L	L
Center loin chops, bone-in, pan-fried	3	L	L
Center loin rib roast, bone-in, lean and fat, roasted	3	L	L
Center loin rib roast, bone-in, roasted	3	L	L
Center loin rib roast, lean and fat, roasted	3	L	L
Center loin rib roast, roasted	3	L	L
Center loin roast, bone-in, lean and fat, roasted	3	L	L
Center loin roast, bone-in, roasted	3	L	L

Unless otherwise stated, all meat is lean and trimmed, and all chops and cutlets are boned. Steaks are medium-sized. Unless otherwise stated, all dishes are homemade.

ENERGY cal	ENERGY J	FAT g	SATURATED FAT g	PROTEIN g	CARBO-HYDRATE g	FIBER g
191	800	11	4	21	0	0
199	832	12	4.3	22	0	0
275	1148	22	8.1	19	0	0
272	1138	21	7.9	19	0	0
291	1216	24	8.6	18	0	0
205	857	13	4.4	21	0	0
275	1148	21	7.8	20	0	0
210	878	13	4.5	23	0	0
229	956	16	5.9	20	0	0
197	825	12	4.4	21	0	0
232	971	13	4.7	26	0	0
193	808	11	3.8	23	0	0
271	1135	18	6.7	24	0	0
220	921	14	5.1	22	0	0
172	718	7	2.6	25	0	0
172	718	7	2.5	26	0	0
210	878	12	4.5	24	0	0
204	853	11	4.1	24	0	0
235	985	14	5.1	25	0	0
197	825	9	3.1	27	0	0
217	907	13	5	23	0	0
190	793	9	3.7	24	0	0
214	896	13	4.5	23	0	0
182	761	9	3	24	0	0
199	832	11	4.3	22	0	0
169	708	8	2.8	23	0	0

PORK, BACON, AND HAM	AVERAGE PORTION oz	GI	GL
Center rib chops, bone-in, braised	3	L	L
Center rib chops, bone-in, broiled	3	L	L
Center rib chops, bone·in, lean and fat, braised	3	L	L
Center rib chops, bone-in, lean and fat, broiled	3	L	L
Center rib chops, bone-in, lean and fat, pan-fried	3	L	L
Center rib chops, bone-in, pan-fried	3	L	L
Center rib chops, braised	3	L	L
Center rib chops, braised	3	L	L
Center rib chops, braised	3	L	L
Center rib chops, broiled	3	L	L
Center rib chops, broiled	3	L	L
Center rib chops, lean and fat, braised	3	L	L
Center rib chops, lean and fat, broiled	3	L	L
Center rib chops, lean and fat, broiled	3	L	L
Center rib chops, lean and fat, pan-fried	3	L	L
Center rib chops, pan-fried	3	L	L
Ham			
Ham, canned	3.2	L	L
Ham, Parma	1	L	L
Ham, premium	2	L	L
Ham, prosciutto	1	L	L
Ham, Serrano	1	L	L
Pork shoulder, cured	3.5	L	L
Loin, whole, braised	3	L	L
Loin, whole, broiled	3	L	L
Loin, whole, lean and fat, braised	3	L	L
Loin, whole, lean and fat, broiled	3	L	L
Loin, whole, lean and fat, roasted	3	L	L
Loin, whole, roasted	3	L	L
Pancetta	1.4	L	L
Ribs, country-style, braised	3	L	L

Unless otherwise stated, all meat is lean and trimmed, and all chops and cutlets are boned. Steaks are medium-sized. Unless otherwise stated, all dishes are homemade.

ENERGY cal	ENERGY J	FAT g	SATURATED FAT g	PROTEIN g	CARBO-HYDRATE g	FIBER g
175	733	8	3.1	24	0	0
186	779	8	2.9	26	0	0
212	889	13	5	23	0	0
224	935	13	4.8	24	0	0
225	943	14	54	22	0	0
185	775	9	3.4	24	0	0
179	751	9	3.4	24	0	0
179	751	9	3.4	24	0	0
179	751	9	3.4	24	0	0
184	768	9	3	25	0	0
184	768	9	3	25	0	0
217	907	13	5.2	22	0	0
221	925	13	4.9	23	0	0
221	925	13	4.9	23	0	0
190	796	10	3.7	24	0	0
190	796	10	3.7	24	0	0
96	404	4	1.4	15	0	0
67	280	3.8	1.3	8.2	3.8	0
74	310	3	1	12	0	0
56	234	2.5	0.8	8.4	0.1	0
96	402	9	1.5	3.8	0.2	0
103	435	4	1 .2	1 7	1	0
173	726	8	2.9	24	0	0
178	747	8	3.1	24	0	0
203	850	12	4.3	23	0	0
206	861	12	4.4	23	0	0
211	882	12	4.6	23	0	0
178	743	8	3	24	0	0
137	572	11.9	1.8	7.2	0.2	0
199	832	12	4.2	22	0	0

PORK, BACON, AND HAM	AVERAGE PORTION oz	GI	GL
Ribs, country-style, lean and fat, braised	3	L	L
Ribs, country-style, lean and fat, roasted	3	L	L
Ribs, country-style, roasted	3	L	L
Shoulder, arm picnic, braised	3	L	L
Shoulder, arm picnic, lean and fat, braised	3	L	L
Shoulder, arm picnic, lean and fat, roasted	3	L	L
Shoulder, arm picnic, roasted	3	L	L
Shoulder, whole, lean and fat, roasted	3	L	L
Shoulder, whole, roasted	3	L	L
Spare ribs, lean and fat, braised	3	L	L
Tenderloin, broiled	3	L	L
Tenderloin, lean and fat, broiled	3	L	L
Tenderloin, lean and fat, roasted	3	L	L
Tenderloin, roasted	3	L	L
Top loin chops, broiled	3	L	L
Top loin chops, lean and fat, broiled	3	L	L
Top loin chops, lean and fat, pan-fried	3	L	L
Top loin chops, pan-fried	3	L	L
Top loin roast, lean and fat, roasted	3	L	L
Top loin roast, roasted	3	L	L
VEAL			
Ground, broiled	3	L	L
Rib, lean and fat, braised	3	L	L
Rib, lean and fat, roasted	3	L	L
Rib, roasted	3	L	L
Shank (fore and hind), braised	3	L	L
Shank (fore and hind), lean and fat, braised	3	L	L
Sirloin, braised	3	L	L
Sirloin, lean and fat, braised	3	L	L
Sirloin, lean and fat, roasted	3	L	L
Sirloin, roasted	3	L	L

Unless otherwise stated, all meat is lean and trimmed, and all chops and cutlets are boned. Steaks are medium-sized. Unless otherwise stated, all dishes are homemade.

ENERGY cal	ENERGY J	FAT g	SATURATED FAT g	PROTEIN g	CARBO-HYDRATE g	FIBER g
252	1052	18	6.8	20	0	0
279	1166	22	7.8	20	0	0
210	878	13	4.5	23	0	0
211	882	10	3.5	27	0	0
280	1170	20	7.2	24	0	0
269	1127	20	7.5	20	0	0
194	811	11	3.7	23	0	0
248	1039	18	6.7	20	0	0
196	818	12	4.1	22	0	0
337	1412	26	9.5	25	0	0
159	665	5	1.9	26	0	0
171	715	7	2.5	25	0	0
147	615	5	1.8	24	0	0
139	583	4	1.4	24	0	0
173	722	7	2.3	26	0	0
195	814	10	3.4	25	0	0
218	914	13	4.5	25	0	0
191	800	9	3.1	26	0	0
192	804	10	3.5	24	0	0
165	690	6	2.2	26	0	0
146	612	6	2.6	21	0	0
213	892	11	4.2	28	0	0
194	811	12	4.6	20	0	0
150	630	6	1.8	22	0	0
150	630	4	1	27	0	0
162	679	5	1.8	27	0	0
173	726	6	1.5	29	0	0
214	896	11	4.4	27	0	0
172	718	9	3.8	21	0	0
143	598	5	2	22	0	0

CHICKEN	AVERAGE PORTION oz	GI	GL
Breast, broiled	4.6	L	L
Breast, broiled and skinned	4.6	L	L
Breast, casseroled	4.6	L	L
Breast, flour-coated, fried	3.5	L	L
Breast, fried in batter	5	L	L
Breast, skinned, broiled	4.6	L	L
Breast, skinned, casseroled	4.6	L	L
Breast, skinned, fried	3	L	L
Breast strips, stir-fried	3.2	L	L
Corn-fed chicken, dark meat, roasted	3.2	L	L
Corn-fed chicken, light meat, roasted	3.2	L	L
Dark meat, flour-coated, fried	3.9	L	L
Dark meat, fried in batter	5.8	L	L
Dark meat, roasted	3.5	L	L
Dark meat, skinned, fried	3.3	L	L
Drumsticks, casseroled	1.7	L	L
Drumsticks, flour-coated, fried	1.8	H	H
Drumsticks, fried in batter	2.6	H	H
Drumsticks, roasted	1.7	L	L
Drumsticks, skinned, casseroled	1.7	L	L
Drumsticks, skinned, fried	1.5	L	L
Drumsticks, skinned, roasted	1.7	L	L
Leg, flour-coated, fried	4	H	H
Leg, fried in batter	5.5	H	H
Leg quarter, casseroled	5.2	L	L
Leg quarter, roasted	5.2	L	L
Leg quarter, skinned, casseroled	5.2	L	L
Leg, skinned, fried	3.3	L	L
Light meat, flour-coated, fried	4.6	H	H
Light meat, fried in batter	4	H	H
Light meat, roasted	3.5	L	L
Light meat, skinned, fried	3.5	L	L
Thighs, casseroled	1.6	L	L
Thighs, flour-coated, fried	2.2	H	H

Unless otherwise stated, chicken and turkey are neither skinned nor boned, game is skinned and trimmed, and dishes are homemade.

ENERGY cal	ENERGY J	FAT g	SATURATED FAT g	PROTEIN g	CARBO- HYDRATE g	FIBER g
225	946	8	1.2	38	0	0
191	807	4	1.2	39	0	0
239	1004	11	3.1	35	0	0
218	910	9	2.4	31	2	0.1
364	1523	18	4.9	35	13	0.4
192	814	4	0.8	42	0	0
148	628	7	2	37	0	0
161	673	4	1.1	29	0	0
145	609	4	0.8	27	0	0
167	695	9	2.5	22	0	0
127	536	4	1.1	23	0	0
314	1311	19	5	30	4	0
498	2082	31	8.3	36	16	0
196	819	11	2.9	24	0	0
217	910	11	2.8	26	2	0
102	425	7	1.8	10	0	0
120	502	7	1.8	13	1	0
193	807	11	3	16	6	0.2
87	364	4	1.2	12	0	0
87	363	5	1.2	11	0	0
82	343	3	0.9	12	0	0
71	301	2	0.7	13	0	0
284	1191	16	4.4	30	3	0.1
431	1804	26	6.8	34	14	0.5
317	1320	20	5.5	33	0	0
345	1432	25	6.7	31	0	0
257	1075	12	3.4	37	0	0
196	818	9	2.3	27	1	0
320	1338	16	4.3	40	2	0.1
313	1310	17	4.7	27	11	0
153	645	4	1	30	0	0
192	803	6	1.5	33	0	0
105	436	7	2	10	0	0
162	680	9	2.5	17	2	0.1

CHICKEN

	AVERAGE PORTION oz	GI	GL
Thighs, fried in batter	3	H	H
Thighs, skinned and boned, casseroled	1.6	L	L
Thighs, skinned, fried	1.9	L	L
Wing quarter, casseroled	5.3	L	L
Wing quarter, skinned, casseroled	5.3	L	L
Wing quarter, roasted	5.3	L	L
Wings, broiled	5.3	L	L
Wings, flour-coated, fried	1.2	H	H
Wings, fried in batter	1.8	H	H
Wings, skinned, fried	0.7	L	L

CHICKEN PRODUCTS AND DISHES

Breaded/battered chicken pieces	3.5	H	H
Breaded chicken strips	3.5	H	H
Chicken and mushroom pie, single crust	3.5	H	H
Chicken curry	12.3	L	L
Chicken curry, with bone	12.3	L	L
Chicken curry, without bone	10.6	L	L
Chicken fingers, baked	3.2	H	H
Chicken goujons, baked	3.2	H	H
Chicken in crumbs, stuffed with cheese and vegetables, baked	3.5	H	H
Chicken in sauce with vegetables	10.2	L	L
Chicken in white sauce, canned	3.5	L	L
Chicken in white sauce, made with low-fat milk	7	L	L
Chicken in white sauce, made with whole milk	7	L	L
Chicken Kiev, frozen, baked	6	H	H
Chicken pie, individual, baked	4.6	H	H
Coated chicken patty, baked	3.5	H	H
Coated chicken steak, baked	3.5	H	H
Curry chicken salad	7	L	L

Unless otherwise stated, chicken and turkey are neither skinned nor boned, game is skinned and trimmed, and dishes are homemade.

ENERGY cal	ENERGY J	FAT g	SATURATED FAT g	PROTEIN g	CARBO-HYDRATE g	FIBER g
238	997	14	3.8	19	8	0.3
81	340	4	1.1	12	0	0
113	474	5	1.4	15	1	0
315	1316	19	5.3	37	0	0
246	1035	9	2.6	40	0	0
339	1415	21	5.9	37	0	0
274	1146	17	4.6	27	Trace	0
103	430	7	1.9	8	1	0
159	664	11	2.9	10	5	0.1
42	177	2	0.5	6	0	0
256	1073	13.9	2.1	14.4	19.6	1.1
277	1161	14	4	19.4	19.6	0.7
200	836	10	4.5	13	14	0.6
522	2174	31	14	42	19	4.5
539	2237	44	6	27	8	2.4
615	2550	51	6.6	31	9	2.7
185	774	9	2.7	11	17	Trace
249	1045	13	3.6	17	18	0.6
230	963	14	4.1	16	11	0.9
336	1412	15	7	39	13	0.9
141	590	8	2.3	14	3	Trace
310	1298	16	5	34	10	0.2
328	1376	18	6.2	34	10	0.2
456	1902	29	12.1	32	19	1
374	1563	21	9.1	12	32	1
266	1113	15.5	2.6	14.2	18.7	1.1
234	982	11.6	1.8	17.7	15.8	1.1
728	3012	63	10.4	33	6	Trace

CHICKEN PRODUCTS AND DISHES

	AVERAGE PORTION oz	GI	GL
Frankfurter, chicken	1.6	L	L
Lemon chicken	3.5	L	L
Tandoori chicken	3.5	L	L

GAME

Bison, roasted	3	L	L
Duck, roasted	6.5	L	L
Duck, untrimmed, roasted	6.5	L	L
Goose, roasted	6.5	L	L
Goose, untrimmed, roasted	6.5	L	L
Venison, roasted	4.2	L	L

TURKEY

Breast, broiled and skinned	3.2	L	L
Dark meat, roasted	3.2	L	L
Drumsticks, roasted	3.2	L	L
Light meat, roasted	3.2	L	L
Thighs, skinned and boned, casseroled	3.2	L	L

TURKEY PRODUCTS

Frankfurter, turkey	1.6	L	L
Louis Rich, honey roasted, fat-free bird	1.8	L	L
Louis Rich, turkey bacon	1	L	L
Louis Rich, turkey bologna	1	L	L
Oscar Mayer, Smokies sausage little	1.9	L	L
Oscar Mayer, wieners	1.9	L	L
Oscar Mayer, wieners	1.6	L	L
Pastrami, turkey	1	L	L
Pot pie, frozen	14	H	H
Salami, turkey	1	L	L
Turkey patties, breaded, battered, fried	2.3	H	H

Unless otherwise stated, chicken and turkey are neither skinned nor boned, game is skinned and trimmed, and dishes are homemade.

ENERGY cal	ENERGY J	FAT g	SATURATED FAT g	PROTEIN g	CARBO-HYDRATE g	FIBER g
116	484	9	2.5	6	3	0
155	652	6	0.8	16	9	Trace
214	897	11	3.3	27	2	Trace
122	508	2	0.8	24	0	0
361	1508	19	6.1	47	0	0
783	3238	92	21.1	37	0	0
590	2455	41	13.7	54	0	0
557	2316	39	12.2	51	0	0
198	838	3	1	43	0	0
140	592	2	0.5	32	0	0
159	671	6	1.8	26	0	0
167	702	8	2.3	25	0	0
138	583	2	0.6	30	0	0
163	684	7	2.3	25	0	0
102	426	8	2.7	6	1	0
57	239	0	0.1	11	3	0
68	286	5	1.5	4	1	0
52	216	4	1.1	3	1	0
172	718	15	5.4	7	1	0
111	463	8	3	7	2	0
145	606	13	4.3	5	1	0
82	342	4	1	11	1	0
699	2922	35	11.4	26	70	4.4
114	476	8	2.3	9	0	0
181	758	12	3	9	10	0.3

FISH	AVERAGE PORTION oz	GI	GL
Anchovies, canned in oil	0.1	L	L
Cod, baked	4.2	L	L
Cod, dried, salted, boiled	3.2	L	L
Cod, frozen, grilled	4.2	L	L
Cod, in batter, fried	6.3	H	H
Cod, in batter, frozen, baked	6.3	H	H
Cod, in breadcrumbs, baked	6.3	H	H
Cod, in parsley sauce, frozen, boiled	6	M	M
Cod, microwaved	4.2	L	L
Cod, poached	4.2	L	L
Cod, smoked, poached	4.2	L	L
Cod, steamed	4.2	L	L
Conger eel, grilled	4	L	L
Dogfish, in batter, fried	4.4	H	H
Haddock, grilled	4.2	L	L
Haddock, in batter, fried	4.2	H	H
Haddock, in breadcrumbs, fried	4.2	H	H
Haddock, in flour, fried	4.2	H	H
Haddock, poached	4.2	L	L
Haddock, smoked, poached	5.3	L	L
Haddock, smoked, steamed	5.3	L	L
Haddock, steamed	4.2	L	L
Hake, grilled	5.2	L	L
Halibut, grilled	5.2	L	L
Halibut, poached	3.9	L	L
Halibut, steamed	3.9	L	L
Herring, grilled	4.2	L	L
Herring, pickled	3.2	L	L
Kipper, baked	6.6	L	L
Kipper, grilled	4.6	L	L
Lemon sole, grilled	3.8	L	L
Lemon sole, steamed	3.8	L	L
Lemon sole, strips, baked	6	H	H
Lemon sole, strips, fried	6	H	H

Unless otherwise stated, values for bottled and canned seafood are for
drained weights. Dishes are homemade unless otherwise stated.

ENERGY cal	ENERGY J	FAT g	SATURATED FAT g	PROTEIN g	CARBO-HYDRATE g	FIBER g
6	24	0.3	0	0.8	0	0
120	510	0.6	0.1	28.7	0	0
124	527	1	0.2	29	0	0
114	482	2	0.5	25	Trace	0
445	1856	28	7.4	29	21	0.9
380	1589	21	6.5	23	26	1.1
367	1544	14.9	2.4	24.7	35.6	3.1
143	598	5	3	20	5	0.2
118	497	0.5	0.1	28.2	0	0
113	475	1	0.4	25	Trace	0
121	511	2	0.7	26	Trace	0
100	420	1	0.2	22	0	0
158	660	6	Trace	25	0	0
369	1531	27	6.6	18	13	0.5
118	500	0.4	0.1	28.7	0	0
278	1163	17	4.4	21	12	0.5
209	875	10	0.8	26	4	0.2
166	698	5	0.5	25	5	0.2
136	572	5	3.1	21	1	0
138	584	0.8	0.1	32.7	0	0
152	644	1	0.3	35	0	0
112	472	0.7	0.1	26.2	0	0
113	478	3	0.4	22	0	0
175	744	3	0.6	37	0	0
169	713	6	3	27	1	0
144	608	4	0.6	26	0	0
215	900	13	3.3	24	0	0
188	789	10	3.3	15	9	0
267	1112	15	2.3	33	0	0
319	1326	22.9	4.9	28.2	0	0
106	445	2	0.2	22	0	0
99	419	1	0.1	22	0	0
318	1318	25	Trace	27	25	Trace
636	2640	49	5.4	26	24	Trace

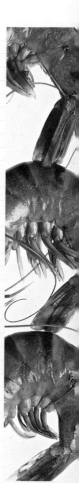

FISH	AVERAGE PORTION oz	GI	GL
Mackerel, canned in brine	1.5	L	L
Mackerel, canned in tomato sauce	4.4	M	L
Mackerel, fried	5.7	L	L
Mackerel, grilled	5	L	L
Mackerel, smoked	5.3	L	L
Monkfish, grilled	2.5	L	L
Mullet, Grey, grilled	3.5	L	L
Mullet, Red, grilled	3.5	L	L
Plaice, frozen, grilled	5.8	L	L
Plaice, frozen, steamed	4.6	L	L
Plaice, goujons, baked	4.6	H	H
Plaice, goujons, fried	5.3	H	H
Plaice, grilled	4.6	L	L
Plaice, in batter, fried	7	H	H
Plaice, in breadcrumbs, baked	5.3	H	H
Plaice, in breadcrumbs, fried	5.3	H	M
Plaice, steamed	4.6	L	L
Red snapper, fried	3.6	L	L
Rock salmon, in batter, fried	4.4	H	H
Salmon, cold smoked	2	L	L
Salmon, grilled/baked	3.5	L	L
Salmon, hot smoked	2	L	L
Salmon, pink, canned in brine, skinned and boned	3.5	L	L
Salmon, raw	3.5	L	L
Salmon, red, canned in brine, skinned and boned	3.5	L	L
Salmon, steamed	2.7	L	L
Sardines, canned in brine	1.5	L	L
Sardines, canned in oil	3.5	L	L
Sardines, canned in tomato sauce	1.5	M	L
Sardines, grilled	1.4	L	L
Sea bass, baked	3.5	L	L
Sea bass, grilled	3.5	L	L

Unless otherwise stated, values for bottled and canned seafood are for
drained weights. Dishes are homemade unless otherwise stated.

ENERGY cal	ENERGY J	FAT g	SATURATED FAT g	PROTEIN g	CARBO-HYDRATE g	FIBER g
92	382	6.3	1.4	8.6	0	0
258	1070	19	4.1	20	2	Trace
438	1819	31	6.4	39	0	0
396	1644	31.4	7.1	28.4	0	0
452	1892	36.2	7.6	31.7	0	0
67	285	0	0.1	16	0	0
150	629	5	1.4	26	0	0
133	561	5	1.4	22	0	0
200	843	3	0.5	42	0	0
120	506	2	0.3	25	0	0
395	1651	24	0	11	36	Trace
639	2657	48	5.4	13	41	Trace
125	525	2	0.4	26	0	0
514	2144	34	9	30	24	1
365	1527	17.4	1.8	21.6	32.3	0.8
342	1427	21	2.3	27	13	0.3
121	510	2	0.4	25	0	0
129	542	3	0.7	25	0	0
369	1531	27	6.6	18	13	0.5
103	431	5.7	1.2	12.8	0.3	0
166	694	7.6	1.3	24	0.5	0
104	435	4.9	1.1	14.2	0.7	0
153	644	7	1.3	24	0	0
180	750	11	1.9	20	0	0
167	700	8	1.7	22	0	0
152	634	10	1.8	15	0	0
77	320	4.1	1.2	4.1	0	0
220	918	14	2.9	23	0	0
79	328	4.9	1.3	8.3	0.4	0
78	326	4	1.2	10	0	0
154	646	6.8	1.5	23.2	0	0
125	524	3	0.7	24	0	0

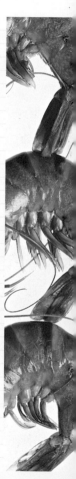

FISH

	AVERAGE PORTION oz	GI	GL
Skate, grilled	7.6	L	L
Skate, in batter, fried	6	H	H
Sole, grilled	4.2	L	L
Swordfish, grilled	4.4	L	L
Trout, brown, steamed	5.5	L	L
Trout, rainbow, baked	5.5	L	L
Trout, rainbow, grilled	5.5	L	L
Tuna, canned in brine	1.5	L	L
Tuna, canned in sunflower oil	1.5	L	L
Tuna, grilled/baked	3.5	L	L
Tuna, raw	1.5	L	L
Whitebait, in flour, fried	2.8	H	H
Whiting, in breadcrumbs, fried	2.7	H	H
Whiting, steamed	3	L	L

FISH PRODUCTS AND DISHES

Fish cakes, breaded, baked	3.5	H	H
Fish cakes, fried	3.5	M	M
Fish cakes, grilled	3.5	H	H
Fish cakes, salmon, breaded, baked	3.5	H	H
Fish cakes, salmon, grilled	3.5	H	H
Fish fingers, cod, fried	2	L	L
Fish fingers, cod, grilled/baked	3.5	H	H
Fish fingers, pollack, grilled	3.5	H	H
Fish fingers, salmon, grilled/baked	3.5	H	H
Fish pie	6	H	H
Kedgeree	10.6	H	H
Salmon en croûte, store bought	3.5	H	H

Unless otherwise stated, values for bottled and canned seafood are for
drained weights. Dishes are homemade unless otherwise stated.

ENERGY cal	ENERGY J	FAT g	SATURATED FAT g	PROTEIN g	CARBO-HYDRATE g	FIBER g
170	725	1	0.2	41	0	0
286	1193	17	4.3	25	8	0.3
109	466	0.7	0.2	25.8	0	0
174	729	6	1.5	29	0	0
209	877	7	1.6	36	0	0
233	977	9.5	2.2	36.9	0	0
209	876	8	1.7	33	0	0
49	205	0.5	0.1	11.2	0	0
72	300	2.9	0.4	11.4	0	0
146	611	4	0.8	27.3	0.4	0
48	204	0.3	0.1	11.3	0	0
420	1739	38	2.1	16	4	0.2
309	1298	17	1.8	29	11	0.3
78	331	1	0.1	18	0	0
206	867	9.4	1	9.3	22.6	0.4
218	912	14	1.4	8	16	0.6
154	650	5	0.6	10	20	0.6
245	1027	13.7	2	11.4	20.4	0.4
273	1137	20	2.9	10	14	0.7
133	557	8	2	7	9	0.3
223	932	9.2	1.2	14.3	22	0.7
213	897	9.2	1.2	13.9	20	1.8
247	1035	11.2	1.1	17.2	20.7	1
210	880	8.2	4.3	11.2	24.5	1
498	2103	24	6.9	43	32	Trace
288	1202	19	3.1	12	18	0.3

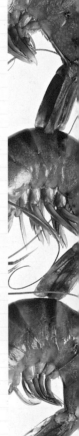

SEAFOOD AND SHELLFISH	AVERAGE PORTION oz	GI	GL
Calamari, grilled/baked	3.5		
Calamari, in batter, fried	4.2	H	H
Clams, breaded and fried	3	H	H
Crab, boiled, dressed with shell	4.6	L	L
Crab, brown meat, cooked	1.8	L	L
Crab, white meat, cooked	1.8	L	L
Langoustines (Dublin Bay prawns), boiled	3.5	L	L
Lobster, boiled, dressed with shell	8.8	L	L
Mussels, boiled and shelled	1.4	L	L
Mussels, canned or bottled without shells	1.4	L	L
Mussels, cooked	3.5	L	L
Oysters, battered or breaded, and fried	5	H	H
Oysters, uncooked and shelled	4.2	L	L
Shrimp, cooked	2	L	L
Shrimp, king, cooked	3.5	L	L
Shrimp, king, grilled	3.5	L	L
Scallops, grilled/baked	3.5	L	L
Scallops, steamed and shelled	2.5	L	L
Shrimp, breaded and fried	3	H	H
Squid, fried	3	H	H

SEAFOOD PRODUCTS AND DISHES			
Clam chowder, Manhattan style, canned, chunky	8.4	L	L
Clam chowder, Manhattan style, canned	8.6	L	L
Clam chowder, New England, canned	8.8	L	L
Clam and tomato juice, canned	5.8	L	L
Mussels in white wine sauce	3.5	L	L
Seafood cocktail	3.1	L	L
Shrimps, canned	3	L	L

Unless otherwise stated, values for bottled and canned seafood are for drained weights. Dishes are homemade unless otherwise stated.

ENERGY cal	ENERGY J	FAT g	SATURATED FAT g	PROTEIN g	CARBO- HYDRATE g	FIBER g
131	548	4.6	1	18.8	3.8	0
234	978	12	2.5	14	19	0.6
172	718	9	2.3	12	9	0.3
166	696	7	0.9	25	Trace	0
73	304	3.9	0.6	9.4	0.5	0
43	180	0.2	0	10.3	0.5	0
86	369	0.8	0.2	0.8	0	0
258	1088	4	0.5	55	Trace	0
42	176	1	0.2	7	1	0
39	166	1	0.2	7	1	0
104	438	2.2	0.3	17.7	0	0
368	1542	18	4.6	13	40	0.3
78	330	2	0.2	13	3	0
42	177	0.5	0.1	9.2	0	0
68	290	0.4	0.1	16.2	0	0
102	433	0.9	0.2	23.5	0	0
127	531	3.9	0.6	20.2	2.9	0
83	351	1	0.3	16	2	Trace
206	861	10	1.8	18	10	0.3
149	622	6	1.6	15	7	0
134	562	3	2.1	7	19	2.9
78	327	2	0.4	2	12	1.5
164	684	7	3	9	17	1.5
80	334	0	0.1	1	18	0.3
81	341	3.2	1.3	9.7	3.7	0.1
77	325	1	0.3	14	3	0
102	427	2	0.3	20	1	0

BURGERS

	AVERAGE PORTION oz	GI	GL
Cheeseburger, large, double patty	9.1	H	H
Cheeseburger, large, single patty	7.7	H	H
Cheeseburger, regular, double patty	8	H	H
Cheeseburger, triple patty, plain	10.6	H	H
Hamburger, large, double patty	7.9	H	H
Hamburger, large, single patty, with condiments	6.1	H	H
Hamburger, large, triple patty, with condiments	9.2	H	H
Hamburger, regular, double patty, plain	6.2	H	H
Hamburger, regular, double patty, with condiments	7.6	H	H
Hamburger, regular, single patty, plain	3.2	H	H
Hamburger, regular, single patty, with condiments	3.8	H	H

PIZZAS

Cheese and tomato, deep pan	7.8	M	H
Cheese and tomato, thin base	4.1	M	H
Meat, deep pan	8.1	M	H
Meat topped, thin base	5.3	M	H
Vegetable, deep pan	10.2	M	H
Pizza, vegetable, thin base	5.3	M	H

FRIED CHICKEN

Deep fried chicken breast, boneless	3.5	H	H
Deep fried chicken drumsticks, bone removed	2.6	H	H
Deep fried chicken thigh, boneless	3.5	H	H
Deep fried chicken wing, bone removed	1.8	H	H
Deep fried coated chicken pieces	3.5	H	H

Unless otherwise stated, burgers include condiments and vegetables, and pizzas are takeout.

ENERGY cal	ENERGY J	FAT g	SATURATED FAT g	PROTEIN g	CARBO-HYDRATE g	FIBER g
704	2946	44	17.7	38	40	2.1
563	2354	33	15	28	38	2.1
650	2718	35	12.8	30	53	2.1
796	3332	51	21.7	56	27	2.1
540	2260	27	10.5	34	40	2.1
427	1785	21	7.9	23	37	2.1
692	2893	41	15.9	50	29	2.1
544	2276	28	10.4	30	43	2
576	2410	32	12	32	39	2.1
274	1148	12	4.1	12	31	2
272	1140	10	3.6	12	34	2.3
547	2310	16	11.4	27	77	4.8
322	1355	12	9.3	17	39	2.2
557	2345	21	14	30	67	4.6
391	1642	18	7.5	21	39	2.8
621	2624	18	7.8	32	88	4.9
332	1398	11	4.1	16	44	2.8
227	949	11.9	2.7	21.9	8.5	0.4
187	785	11.3	3	15.8	6	0.2
231	969	14.2	3.6	18.6	7.8	0.3
156	652	10.7	2.6	9.8	5.4	0.2
233	972	12.8	3.1	24.8	4.8	0.8

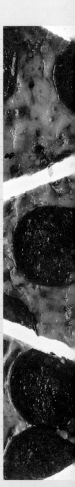

MISCELLANEOUS	AVERAGE PORTION oz	GI	GL
Corndog	6.1	M	H
Hotdog, plain	3.4	H	H
Hotdog, with chili	4	H	H
Hotdog, with onions, ketchup, and relish	3.5	H	H
Hush puppies	2.7	H	H
Pancakes with butter and syrup	8.1	H	H
MEXICAN DISHES			
Burrito, beans	7.6	L	L
Burrito, beans and cheese	6.5	L	L
Burrito, beans and chili peppers	7.1	L	L
Burrito, beans and meat	8	L	L
Burrito, beans, cheese, and beef	7.1	L	L
Burrito, beef	7.6	L	L
Burrito, beef and chili peppers	7	L	L
Burrito, beef, cheese, and chili peppers	10.6	L	L
Chimichanga, beef	6.1	L	L
Chimichanga, beef and cheese	6.4	H	H
Chimichanga, beef and chili peppers	6.7	H	H
Chimichanga, beef, cheese, and chili peppers	6.3	H	H
Enchilada, cheese	5.7	M	M
Enchilada, cheese and beef	6.7	M	M
Enchilada, vegetable	12.7	M	M
Fajita, beef with vegetables	7	L	L
Fajita, chicken, meat only	6	L	L
Fajita, chicken with vegetables	8.8	L	L
Nachos, cheese	6	H	H
Nachos, cheese and jalapeno peppers	7.1	H	H
Nachos, cheese, beans, ground beef, and peppers	9	H	H
Tacos/Tostada, beans and cheese	5.1	M	H
Tacos/Tostada, beans, beef, and cheese	7.9	M	H
Tacos/Tostada, beef and cheese	5.7	M	H

Unless otherwise specified, burgers include garnish, seasonings, and sauce.

ENERGY cal	ENERGY J	FAT g	SATURATED FAT g	PROTEIN g	CARBO-HYDRATE g	FIBER g
460	1925	19	5.2	17	56	1
242	1012	15	5.1	10	18	1
296	1240	13	4.9	14	31	1
215	903	9.3	2.3	7.1	27.4	1.8
257	1074	12	2.7	5	35	1.5
520	2174	14	5.9	8	91	1
447	1871	13	6.9	14	71	1.5
378	1579	12	6.8	15	55	1.5
412	1724	15	7.6	16	58	1.5
508	2125	18	8.3	22	66	1.5
331	1384	13	7.1	15	40	1.5
524	2191	21	10.5	27	59	1.5
426	1783	17	8	22	49	1.5
632	2645	25	10.4	41	64	1.5
425	1777	20	8.5	20	43	1.5
443	1854	23	11.2	20	39	1.5
424	1773	19	8.3	18	46	1.5
364	1521	18	8.4	15	38	1.5
319	1337	19	10.6	10	29	1
323	1350	18	9	12	30	1
525	1690	26	7.6	23	54	7.6
420	1757	15.4	7.8	23.2	50.2	4.2
213	676	11	3.6	29	1	1.7
453	1895	12.8	2.8	24.9	63.4	2.9
438	1208	31	11.6	18	24	3.4
608	2544	34	14	17	60	2
569	2379	31	12.5	20	56	2
223	935	10	5.4	10	27	1.5
333	1393	17	11.5	16	30	1.5
315	1317	16	10.4	19	23	1.5

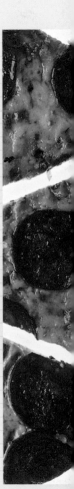

MEXICAN DISHES	AVERAGE PORTION oz	GI	GL
Tacos/Tostada, chicken and vegetables	3.5	M	H
Tacos/Tostada, beef and vegetables	3.5	M	H

INDIAN DISHES			
Bombay aloo	3.5	H	H
Chicken biryani	14	H	H
Chicken, butter/murgh makhani	12.3	L	L
Chicken dhansak	12.3	L	L
Chicken jalfrezi	12.3	L	L
Chicken korma	12.3	L	L
Chicken madras	12.3	L	L
Chicken tikka	12.3	L	L
Chicken vindaloo	12.3	L	L
Lamb balti	12.3	L	L
Lamb ragan josh	12.3	L	L
Naan bread	1.8	M	H
Poppadoms	2.5	M	H
Raita	1.8	L	L
Saag paneer	12.3	L	L
Samosa, meat	2.5	H	H
Vegetable balti	12.3	L	L
Vegetable bhaji	3.5	H	H
Vegetable biryani	12.3	H	H

SOUTH-EAST ASIAN DISHES			
Aromatic crispy duck	4.4	L	L
Barbecue pork bun	3.5	H	H
Barbecue roast pork	3.5	L	L
California roll	3.5	H	H
Cantonese egg tart	1.8	M	H
Chicken chop suey, thick sauce	15.9	M	M
Chicken chow mein	12.3	H	H

Unless otherwise specified, pizzas are takeout.

ENERGY cal	ENERGY J	FAT g	SATURATED FAT g	PROTEIN g	CARBO-HYDRATE g	FIBER g
178	746	8.9	3	12.8	12.5	1.8
279	1168	16.2	5	13.9	20.7	2.7
118	492	6.7	0.8	2	13.8	1.2
651	2144	30	8	34	66	4.4
666	2786	50.4	26.3	45.5	18.6	3.5
503	1509	30	6	40	21	6.7
416	1203	27	5.3	34	11	7
668	1753	51	20	44	8	7
408	1707	22	9.8	44.4	9.4	7.8
421	1470	15	5.6	71	Trace	1
424	1782	14.3	2.6	68.6	9.5	1.1
534	1518	35	8.8	43	11	6.7
510	1422	35	9.8	43	6	3.1
142	602	3.6	0.5	3.9	25.1	1
351	916	27	5.6	8	20	4.1
57	241	2.2	1.5	4.2	5.8	0.7
412	1723	18.8	6	12.1	51.7	7.7
191	553	12	3.2	8	13	1.5
373	983	28	5.3	8	23	7.7
166	688	13.7	1.5	3.4	8.2	1.9
467	1468	25	4.9	10	55	6
412	1107	30	9.1	35	15	1.1
273	1143	9.9	3.2	9.4	39	1.4
207	867	13.4	5.5	18.8	3	0.4
116	485	0.5	0.1	5.3	24.3	0.9
41	172	2.3	0.9	0.7	4.7	0.1
363	1095	21	3.6	37	7	5.4
516	1662	25	4.2	30	46	3.9

SOUTH-EAST ASIAN DISHES	AVERAGE PORTION oz	GI	GL
Chicken fried rice	12.3	H	H
Chicken satay	6	L	L
Chicken with cashew nuts	12.7	L	L
Chinese roast duck with skin	3.5	L	L
Egg fried rice	9.5	H	H
Green chicken curry	12.3	L	L
Meat spring roll	1.9	H	H
Salmon maki	3.5	H	H
Salmon nigiri sushi	3.5	H	H
Sesame shrimp toasts	2.5	H	H
Shrimp crackers	2.5	M	M
Spare ribs	12	L	L
Steamed barbecue pork bun	1.8	H	H
Steamed chicken bun	1.8	H	H
Steamed pork dumpling ("siu mai")	1	L	L
Steamed shrimp dumpling ("har gow")	1	L	L
Steamed rice roll with barbecue pork	3.5	H	H
Steamed rice roll with shrimp	3.5	H	H
Steamed sticky rice	3.5	H	H
Stir-fried beef with green peppers in black bean sauce	12.7	L	L
Stir-fried chicken with vegetables	7	L	L
Stir-fried Thai vegetable curry	12.3	L	L
Stir-fried vegetables	12	L	L
Sweet and sour chicken	10.6	M	M
Szechuan shrimp with vegetables	12.3	L	L
Thai red chicken curry	12.3	L	L
Tuna maki	3.5	H	H
Tuna nigiri sushi	3.5	H	H
Vegetable maki	3.5	H	H
Wonton, deep fried	1	M	M
Wonton noodles in soup	8	H	H

Unless otherwise specified, pizzas are takeout.

ENERGY cal	ENERGY J	FAT g	SATURATED FAT g	PROTEIN g	CARBO-HYDRATE g	FIBER g
562	1948	21	3.5	23	75	0
324	1006	18	4.9	37	5	3.7
470	1331	31	5.4	38	10	0
332	1388	28.4	9.6	19	0	0
491	1809	13	1.6	12	87	2.2
417	1125	30	18.2	31	5	8.4
133	374	9	2.1	4	10	1
167	699	1.6	0.3	7.4	32.8	0.5
180	753	5.7	1.1	8.7	25.2	0.7
268	699	21	2.7	9	12	1.3
386	1061	27	2.6	0	37	0.8
873	2358	64	10.2	75	7	1
129	539	3.7	0.9	3.7	21.5	0.4
108	451	3	0.8	3.8	17.5	1
60	249	3.9	1.1	3.3	3	0.4
46	194	2	0.5	2	5.4	0
139	583	5.7	1.6	5.1	18	1
99	415	2.2	0.4	3.9	17	0
208	869	7.3	2.4	6.4	31	1
373	1158	20	5	38	11	6.5
248	1046	8.4	1.5	38.2	5.4	1.2
351	882	29	13.7	13	11	9.1
177	455	14	2.4	6	7	6.1
575	1810	30	3.9	23	57	1.8
297	912	16	1.8	27	11	4.9
286	1196	8.5	2.3	19.7	35	7.1
158	661	0.4	0.1	7.8	32.8	0.5
153	640	0.7	0.2	8.4	30.1	0.7
150	628	1.3	0.1	3.2	33.6	1.2
125	522	8.7	1.3	2.9	9.3	0.4
155	650	5	1.2	11.7	16.9	0.5

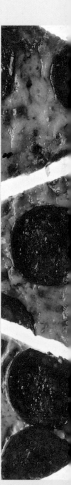

RICE, PASTA, AND NOODLES	AVERAGE PORTION oz	GI	GL
Basmati rice, boiled	8.1	M	H
Brown rice, boiled	6.3	M	H
Bulgur wheat, cooked	3.5	M	M
Couscous, cooked	3.5	M	M
Macaroni, boiled	8.1	L	H
Macaroni, whole-wheat, boiled	8.1	L	H
Millet, cooked	3.5	M	H
Noodles, boiled	8.1	M	H
Noodles, egg, boiled	8.1	M	H
Noodles, fried	8.1	M	H
Noodles, rice, boiled	8.1	M	H
Noodles, soba, boiled	3.5	L	H
Noodles, udon, boiled	3.5	M	H
Pasta, fresh egg, boiled	8.1	L	H
Pasta twists/Italian fusilli, boiled	8.1	M	H
Polenta, boiled	3.5	M	H
Red rice, boiled	8.1	M	H
Risotto rice, boiled	3.5	M	H
Quinoa, cooked	3.5	M	M
Savory rice, cooked	6.3	H	H
Semolina, cooked	3.5	L	H
Short grain rice, boiled	3.5	H	H
Spaghetti, boiled	8.1	L	H
Spaghetti, whole-wheat, boiled	8.1	L	H
White rice, easy cook, boiled	6.3	H	H
White rice, fried in lard/drippings	10.6	H	H
White rice, glutinous, boiled	8.1	H	H
White rice, polished, boiled	8.1	H	H
Whole-wheat pasta, boiled	8.1	L	H
Wild rice, boiled	3.5	L	H

Unless otherwise stated, all dishes are homemade.

ENERGY cal	ENERGY J	FAT g	SATURATED FAT g	PROTEIN g	CARBO-HYDRATE g	FIBER g
405	1698	1.4	0.2	12.9	91.1	1.4
254	1075	2	0.5	5	58	1.4
153	640	0.4	0.1	5.6	33.8	8.2
104	435	0.2	0	3.8	23.2	1.4
198	840	1	0.2	7	43	2.1
198	840	1	0.2	7	43	6.4
112	467	1	0.2	3.5	23.6	1.3
143	607	1	0.2	6	30	1.6
382	1599	2.3	0.5	13.3	82.1	5.1
352	1467	26	1	4	26	1.2
205	860	0.5	0.2	4.4	49	1.6
102	425	0.1	0	5.1	21.4	1.4
131	548	0.5	0	3.5	30	1
350	1467	3.7	0.9	13.3	70.4	2.1
336	1408	0.9	0.2	11	75.7	6.2
40	169	0.2	0	1	9.2	0.9
184	784	1	0.2	4	43	1.4
327	1370	0.4	0.3	7.5	78.3	1.1
139	583	2.2	0.2	5	26.5	2.3
256	1078	6	2	5	47	2.5
104	435	0.3	0.1	4	22.7	1.2
119	498	0.2	0.1	2.4	28.7	0.3
325	1359	1.4	0.5	10.1	72.5	3.5
260	1116	2	0.2	11	53	8.1
248	1057	2	0.5	5	56	0.2
393	1662	10	4.2	7	75	1.8
150	633	1	0.2	4	34	0.5
283	1201	1	0.2	5	68	0.5
308	1289	2.5	0.5	12	63.3	10.1
99	413	0.3	0.1	4	21.3	1.8

RICE AND PASTA DISHES	AVERAGE PORTION oz	GI	GL
Cannelloni, meat, store bought	9.2	H	H
Cannelloni, spinach	12	H	H
Cannelloni, vegetable	12	H	H
Chicken risotto	12	H	H
Fresh egg pasta filled with cheese, store bought, cooked	8.8	L	M
Fresh egg pasta filled with cheese and tomato, store bought, cooked	8.8	L	M
Fresh egg pasta filled with meat, store bought, cooked	8.8	L	M
Fresh egg pasta filled with mushrooms, store bought, cooked	8.8	L	M
Fresh egg pasta filled with vegetables, and cheese, store bought, cooked	8.8	L	M
Lasagne, meat, store bought	14.8	H	H
Lasagne, spinach	14.8	H	H
Lasagne, spinach, whole-wheat	14.8	H	H
Lasagne, vegetable	14.8	H	H
Lasagne, vegetable, whole-wheat	14.8	H	H
Pasta with ham and mushroom sauce	8.3	H	H
Pasta with meat and tomato sauce	8.3	H	H
Pilaff, vegetable	6.3	H	H
Ravioli, canned in tomato sauce	8.8	H	H
Ravioli, stuffed with cheese, tomato and herbs, store bought	8.8	H	H
Ravioli, stuffed with meat and vegetables, store bought	8.8	H	H
Rice and blackeyed beans	7	H	H
Rice and blackeyed beans, brown rice	7	H	H
Risotto, vegetable	10.2	H	H
Spaghetti and meat sauce	14	H	H
Spaghetti, canned in tomato sauce	8.8	H	H
Vine leaves, stuffed with rice	2.8	M	H

Unless otherwise stated, all dishes are homemade.

ENERGY cal	ENERGY J	FAT g	SATURATED FAT g	PROTEIN g	CARBO-HYDRATE g	FIBER g
315	1326	13	5.2	17	35	3.1
449	1880	26	7.8	15	43	2.7
493	2067	31	11.6	15	43	2.4
546	2310	10	4.5	31	84	Trace
539	2256	16.8	8.8	26.3	75.5	5.3
483	2023	14.8	8.3	21.8	70.3	4
500	2094	11.8	4.5	25.3	78.3	3.5
432	1808	10.8	6	20.3	67.8	4.3
487	2037	14.5	8	21.8	71.8	4
601	2533	26	11.8	31	66	2.9
365	1541	13	5.5	15	53	4.6
391	1659	13	5.5	18	55	9.7
428	1810	18	9.2	17	52	4.2
445	1877	19	9.2	20	52	8.8
284	1194	14	8.2	13	27	2.1
263	1102	10	4	16	30	2
248	1053	8	4.3	5	43	1
193	809	3.5	1.3	5.8	37	4
304	1267	13	7.9	17	30	0.6
324	1350	15	8.9	16	34	3.4
366	1556	7	3	12	68	2.8
350	1488	7	3	11	66	3.6
426	1798	19	2.9	12	56	6.4
532	2224	24.8	8.6	24.8	49.6	3.6
180	752	0.8	0.3	5.3	40.5	3.3
210	875	14	2.1	2	19	1

BREAD AND CAKES	AVERAGE PORTION oz	GI	GL
Bagel, cinnamon and raisin	3.5	H	H
Bagel, multigrain	3.5	H	H
Bagel, plain	3.5	H	H
Bagel, poppyseed, onion, sesame	3.5	H	H
Banana bread, homemade	3	H	H
Brioche	1.6	H	H
Brown bread, sliced	1.3	H	L
Brown rolls	1.7	M	L
Cake bar, chocolate	3.5	H	H
Cake bar, plain	3.5	H	H
Cake from "healthy eating" range	0.8	H	H
Cake with jam and butter icing	2	H	H
Caramel shortbread	1.8	H	H
Campione d'Italia garlic bread, frozen	1	H	H
Carrot cake, un-iced, homemade	3	H	H
Carrot cake, iced, store bought	3.5	H	H
Cheese-topped rolls, white	3	H	H
Chocolate cake	1.4	H	H
Chocolate cake, with butter icing	2.2	H	H
Chocolate cake, with filling and icing	3.5	H	H
Chocolate fudge cake	3.4	H	H
Ciabatta, plain	1.8	H	H
Cinnamon-raisin loaf	1.2	H	H
Coconut cake	1.4	M	H
Cornbread, made with low-fat (2%) milk	2.3	H	H
Cupcake, chocolate, un-frosted	3.5	H	H
Cupcake, chocolate, with frosting	3.5	H	H
Cupcake, plain, un-frosted	3.5	H	H
Cupcake, plain, with frosting	3.5	H	H
Danish pastries	3.9	H	H
Doughnuts, cake-type, chocolate, sugared or glazed	1.5	H	H
Doughnuts, cake-type, plain	1.7	H	H

ENERGY cal	ENERGY J	FAT g	SATURATED FAT g	PROTEIN g	CARBO-HYDRATE g	FIBER g
262	1095	1.7	0.3	9.8	55.2	2.3
254	1063	1.3	0.2	11.3	52.5	7.3
273	1161	1.8	0.4	10	57.8	2.4
269	1125	1.8	0.4	11	55.6	2.4
230	968	9	5.6	4	35	1.5
144	607	4	2.8	4	24	1
75	317	1	0.2	3	15	1.3
113	482		2	0.3	5	22
1.8	430	1800	21.6	9.9	5	57.5
355	1485	12.2	5	3.1	62	0.6
61	262	0.6	0.3	0.8	14.1	0.4
213	896	8.9	4.2	2.2	33.1	0.8
233	974	13.7	7.6	2.4	26.8	0.7
101	424	5	0.8	2	12	1.3
349	1454	25	6.4	5	28	2.1
374	1569	20.2	5.1	4.2	46.8	1.1
241	1016	7	3.4	9	38	1.2
182	763	11	8.2	3	20	0.5
313	1306	19	14.3	4	33	0.8
413	1730	23.7	9.5	4.5	48.6	1.8
351	1479	14	4.5	5	55	0.9
135	574	2	0.3	5	26	1.2
18	76	1	0.2	3	0	0.9
174	726	10	2.6	3	20	1
173	723	5	1	4	28	1
333	1396	12.5	2.8	5.8	52.7	1.7
370	1550	14.5	2.9	3.4	60.3	0.8
306	1283	9.3	1.6	4.6	54.5	0.8
355	1485	11.4	2.6	3.1	63.9	0.4
491	2047	32.1	13	5.3	48	1.7
175	733	8	2.2	2	24	0.9
198	828	11	1.7	2	23	0.7

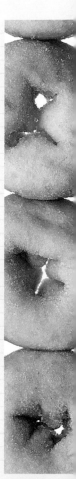

BREAD AND CAKES	AVERAGE PORTION oz	GI	GL
Doughnuts, cake-type, plain, chocolate-coated or frosted	1.5	H	H
Doughnuts, cake-type, plain, sugared, or glazed	1.6	H	H
Doughnuts, cake-type, wheat, sugared or glazed	1.9	H	H
Doughnuts, french crullers, glazed	1.5	H	H
Doughnuts, yeast-leavened, glazed	2	H	H
Doughnuts, yeast-leavened, creme-filled	3	H	H
Doughnuts, yeast-leavened, jelly-filled	3	H	H
English Eccles cakes	1.6	H	H
English mince pies	1.9	H	H
English-style Madeira cake, iced	3	M	H
Focaccia, herb/garlic and coriander	1.8	H	M
French baguette, white	1.4	H	M
French baguette, white, part baked	1.4	H	M
French loaf, multigrain	1.4	M	M
French ficelle, white	1.4	H	M
French/Vienna bread	1	H	M
French/Vienna bread, toasted	1	H	M
Fruit cake	1.6	M	H
Fruit pies, small	1.9	M	H
Garlic and herb baguette	1.4	H	M
Garlic bread	0.7	H	M
Gingerbread	1.8	H	M
Jelly roll	1	H	H
Italian bread	1	H	M
Light white bread, sliced	0.7	H	M
Macarons, with chocolate ganache filling	1	H	H
Muffins, blueberry, homemade with low-fat (2%) milk	2	M	M
Muffins, blueberry, store bought	2	M	M
Muffins, blueberry, toasting, toasted	1.1	M	M
Muffins, chocolate	3.5	M	M

ENERGY cal	ENERGY J	FAT g	SATURATED FAT g	PROTEIN g	CARBO- HYDRATE g	FIBER g	
204	853	13	3.5	2	21	0.9	
192	802	10	2.7	2	23	0.7	
194	813	10	1.6	3	23	1.2	
169	707	8	1.9	1	24	0.5	
226	944	13	3.3	4	25	0.7	
307	1284	21	4.6	5	26	0.7	
289	1210	16	4.1	5	33	0.7	
164	689	8.2	4.2	2	22	0.9	
207	873	8.2	3.3	2.1	33.4	0.9	
312	1312	13.4	5.3	4.1	46.7	1.6	
147	620	4	0.6	5	26	0.7	
109	465	1	0.1	4	24	1	
108	458	1	0.1	4	23	1	
110	467	1	0.1	4	22	1	
101	431	1	0.1	4	21	1	
77	321	1	0.2	2	15	0.8	
86	362	1	0.2	3	16	1	
150	633	5.4	2.1	2	24.8	1.1	
195	821	7.4	2.6	1.7	32.4	0.9	
139	584	6.7	3.5	2.8	18	0.3	
73	306	4	1.9	2	9	1	
190	799	6	1.9	3	32	0.6	
83	352	1	0.3	2	17	0.2	
76	318	1	0.2	2	14	0.8	
46	193	1	0.1	2	9	0.5	
151	630	7.8	1.6	3.2	18	0	
162	679	6	1.2	4	23	1.5	
158	661	4	0.8	3	27	1.5	
103	432	3	0.5	2	18	0.6	
436	1826	25.4	4.8	5.5	49.5	0.8	

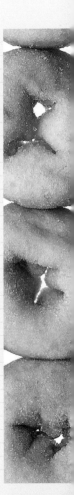

BREAD AND CAKES	AVERAGE PORTION oz	GI	GL
Muffins, corn, homemade with low-fat (2%) milk	2	H	H
Muffins, corn, store bought	2	H	H
Muffins, corn, toasting, toasted	1.3	H	H
Muffins, English, multigrain	2.3	H	H
Muffins, English, plain, enriched	2	H	H
Muffins, English, plain, unenriched	2	H	H
Muffins, English, raisin-cinnamon, apple-cinnamon	2	H	H
Muffins, English, wheat	2	H	H
Muffins, English, wholewheat	2.3	M	M
Muffins, fruit/plain	3.5	H	H
Muffins, oatbran	2	M	M
Muffins, plain, homemade with low-fat (2%) milk	2	H	H
Muffins, wheatbran with raisins, toasting, toasted	1.2	M	M
Multigrain bread, sliced	1.3	L	L
Multigrain rolls	56	L	L
Naan bread, garlic and coriander/plain	5.6	H	M
Oatmeal bread	1	L	L
Oatmeal bread, reduced-calorie	0.7	L	L
Pepperidge Farm crusty Italian garlic bread	1.8	H	H
Pita bread, white	2.6	M	L
Pound cake	1.4	H	H
Pumpernickel bread	1.1	L	L
Rolls, hamburger or hotdog, multigrain	1.5	M	M
Rolls, hamburger or hotdog, plain	1.5	H	H
Rolls, hamburger or hotdog, reduced-calorie	1.5	H	H
Sandwich bread, white	0.5	H	H
Scones, cheese	1.7	H	H
Scones, fruit	1.7	H	H

ENERGY cal	ENERGY J	FAT g	SATURATED FAT g	PROTEIN g	CARBO-HYDRATE g	FIBER g
180	754	7	1.3	4	25	1.9
174	727	5	0.8	3	29	1.9
114	478	4	0.6	2	19	0.5
155	649	1	0.2	6	31	1.8
134	560	1	0.1	4	26	1 .5
134	560	1	0.1	4	26	1.5
139	580	2	0.2	4	28	1.7
127	532	1	0.2	5	26	2.6
134	560	1	0.2	6	27	4.4
375	1569	19.5	2.4	5	47.8	1
154	644	4	0.6	4	28	2.6
169	706	6	1.2	4	24	1.5
106	445	3	0.5	2	19	2.8
87	369	1	0.3	4	18	1.3
133	565	2	0.3	6	24	2
456	1929	12	1.6	12	80	3.2
73	304	1	0.2	2	13	1.1
48	202	1	0.1	2	10	1.1
186	779	10	2.4	4	21	1.3
191	813	1	0.7	7	41	1.8
157	661	6	3.5	2	23	0.4
67	283	1	0.1	2	15	2.1
113	473	3	0.6	4	19	1.6
123	515	2	0.5	4	22	1.2
84	353	1	0.1	4	18	2.7
36	153	1	0.2	1	7	0.3
174	731	9	4.9	5	21	0.8
152	640	5	1.6	4	25	0.8

BREAD AND CAKES	AVERAGE PORTION oz	GI	GL
Scones, plain	1.7	H	H
Scones, whole-wheat	1.8	H	H
Scones, whole-wheat, fruit	1.8	H	H
Sourdough bread	3.5	L	M
Sponge cake, fat-free	2	M	M
Sponge cake, frozen	2	M	M
Sponge cake, with buttercream frosting	2	M	M
Strawberry tartlets	1.8	H	H
Swiss cake rolls, chocolate, individual	1	M	H
Tortilla, wheat, soft	5.6	M	L
Waffles	2.2	H	H
Wheatgerm bread	1	M	L
White bread, crusty bloomer	1.2	H	M
White bread, farmhouse, large	1.2	H	M
White bread, farmhouse, small	0.9	H	M
White bread, premium	1.2	H	M
White bread, standard	1.2	H	M
White bread, standard, toasted	1.2	H	M
White rolls, crusty	1.8	H	M
White rolls, soft	1.6	H	M
Whole-wheat bread	1.3	M	L
Whole-wheat bread, toasted	1.3	M	L
Whole-wheat rolls	1.7	M	L

SANDWICHES			
Bacon, lettuce, and tomato, white bread	7	H	H
Cheese and pickle, white bread	7	H	H
Chicken salad, white bread	7	H	H
Egg mayonnaise, white bread	7	H	H
Ham salad, white bread	7	H	H
Shrimp cocktail/mayonnaise, white bread	7	H	H
Tuna mayonnaise, white bread	7	H	H

ENERGY cal	ENERGY J	FAT g	SATURATED FAT g	PROTEIN g	CARBO- HYDRATE g	FIBER g
166	701	5.9	3.1	3.4	26.5	1.1
163	684	7	2.4	4	22	2.6
162	683	6	2	4	24	2.5
257	1075	3	0.6	8.8	51.9	3
171	722	4	1	6	31	0.5
190	795	10	3.1	2	24	0.4
294	1228	18	5.6	3	31	0.4
111	466	6	3.2	1	14	0.6
124	520	6.8	3.5	1.4	15.3	0.5
451	1903	14	2.9	12	73	3
217	911	11	4.7	6	26	1
66	281	1	0.2	3	12	1.2
86	368	1	0.2	3	18	0.8
83	353	1	0.2	3	17	0.7
66	281	1	0.2	2	14	0.7
83	352	1	0.2	3	17	0.7
79	335	1	0.1	3	17	0.7
97	414	1	0.1	3	21	0
131	558	1	0.3	5	27	1.2
114	485	1	0.3	4	23	0.9
82	349	1	0.2	4	16	1.9
102	431	1	0.2	5	20	0
117	498	2	0.2	5	22	2.1
470	1966	24.8	5.6	16.4	48.2	2.4
579	2426	29.8	14.8	24	57.4	2.2
351	1467	10.6	2.3	21.4	45.2	2.2
248	1040	12	2.4	8.4	28.5	1.2
334	1399	9	1.9	16.4	50	2.4
469	1963	25.4	2.1	19.2	43.6	4.2
476	1991	21	3.5	24.2	50.6	2

CHEESE	AVERAGE PORTION oz	GI	GL
Brie, without rind	1.4	L	L
Camembert	1.4	L	L
Cheddar, English, white	1.4	L	L
Cheddar, half-fat (15% fat)	1.4	L	L
Cheddar, vegetarian	1.4	L	L
Cheese spread	1	L	L
Cheshire, white	1.4	L	L
Cottage (4% fat)	1.4	L	L
Cottage, low-fat (1.5–2% fat)	1.4	L	L
Danish Blue	1	L	L
Dolcelatte, without rind	1.4	L	L
Double Gloucester	1.4	L	L
Edam	1.4	L	L
Emmental	1.4	L	L
Fontina	0.9	L	L
Fromage frais, fruit	3.5	G	L
Fromage frais, fruit, virtually fat-free	3.5	L	L
Fromage frais, natural	3.5	L	L
Fromage frais, natural, virtually fat-free	3.5	L	L
Goat	1.9	L	L
Gouda	1.4	L	L
Halloumi	1.4	L	L
Lancashire	1.4	L	L
Mascarpone	1.9	L	L
Monterey Jack	0.9	L	L
Mozzarella, fresh	1.9	L	L
Mozzarella, grated	1.9	L	L
Paneer	1.4	L	L
Parmesan, drums, freshly grated	0.7	L	L
Parmesan, wedges, freshly grated	0.7	L	L
Pecorino	0.9	L	L
Port Salut	1.4	L	L
Processed cheese, slices	0.7	L	L
Provolone	0.9	L	L

Unless otherwise specified, generic cheeses are made with cows' milk.

ENERGY cal	ENERGY J	FAT g	SATURATED FAT g	PROTEIN g	CARBO-HYDRATE g	FIBER g
144	596	12	7.3	8	2	0
116	482	9	6	9	Trace	0
166	690	14	8.7	10	0	0
109	456	6	4.3	13	Trace	0
156	647	13	8.3	10	Trace	0
81	335	7	4.7	3	2	0
152	630	13	8.5	9	Trace	0
36	149	2	0.9	5	0	0
28	118	1	0.4	5	0	0
103	425	9	5.7	6	Trace	0
158	652	14	8.7	7	Trace	0
165	684	14	9.3	10	Trace	0
136	566	10	6.3	11	Trace	0
160	663	12	8.2	12	Trace	0
110	462	9	5.4	7	0	0
135	566	5.6	0	5.2	16.9	0.4
50	211	0.2	0	6.7	5.6	0.4
113	468	8	5.6	6	4.4	Trace
48	205	0.1	0	7.5	4.6	Trace
174	722	14	9.8	12	Trace	0
151	625	12	8.1	10	Trace	0
124	516	9	6.6	10	0	0
153	633	13	8.4	10	Trace	0
230	949	24	16.2	3	Trace	0
107	443	30	5.4	25	0	0
141	587	11	7.6	10	Trace	0
164	680	12	8.1	14	Trace	0
130	539	10	6.2	10	Trace	0
97	403	7	4.6	9	Trace	0
82	343	6	3.9	7	Trace	0
110	459	8	4.8	1	1	0
133	554	10	7.2	10	Trace	0
59	244	5	2.8	4	1	0
99	417	8	4.8	7	1	0

CHEESE	AVERAGE PORTION oz	GI	GL
Red Leceister	1.4	L	L
Ricotta	1.9	L	L
Romano	0.9	L	L
Roquefort	0.9	L	L
Soft white spreadable, low-fat (<10%)	1	L	L
Soft white spreadable, reduced-fat (15%)	1	L	L
Soft white spreadable, full-fat	1	L	L
St. Paulin	1.4	L	L
Stilton, blue	1.2	L	L
Wensleydale	1.4	L	L

CREAM AND SUBSTITUTES			
Cream, clotted	1.6	L	L
Cream, heavy	1	L	L
Cream, light	0.5	L	L
Cream, sour	1	L	L
Cream, whipping	1	L	L
Cream, frozen, whipping	1	L	L
Cream, sterilized, canned	1.6	L	L
Cream, UHT, canned spray	0.4	L	L
Cream, UHT, half-and-half	0.5	L	L
Cream, UHT, light	15	L	L
Cream, UHT, whipping	1	L	L
Crème fraîche	1.2	L	L
Crème fraîche, low-fat	1.2	L	L
Half-and-half	1	L	L
Non-dairy, whipping	1	L	L

Unless otherwise specified, generic cheeses are made with cows' milk and cream is fresh.

ENERGY cal	ENERGY J	FAT g	SATURATED FAT g	PROTEIN g	CARBO-HYDRATE g	FIBER g
161	667	13	8.9	10	Trace	0
79	329	6	3.8	5	1	0
110	459	8	4.8	1	1	0
105	438	9	5.4	6	1	0
43	182	2	1.7	4	1	0
56	231	5	3.4	3	Trace	0
94	386	9	6.7	2	Trace	0
133	554	10	7.2	10	Trace	0
143	594	12	8.1	8	Trace	0
152	632	13	8.5	9	Trace	0
264	1086	29	17.9	1	1	0
135	555	16	9	1	1	0
30	123	3	1.8	0	1	0
62	254	6	3.8	1	1	0
112	462	12	7.4	1	1	0
114	468	12	7.5	1	1	0
108	443	11	6.7	1	2	0
31	127	2	2	0	0	0
21	86	2	1.2	0	1	0
29	122	3	1.8	0	1	0
112	462	12	7.4	1	1	0
190	792	20	13.2	1.2	1.4	0
85	355	7.5	4.5	1.8	2.5	0
44	184	4	2.5	1	1	0
96	395	9	8.4	1	1	0

EGGS

	AVERAGE PORTION OZ	GI	GL
Battery eggs, raw	2	L	L
Boiled	1.8	L	L
Duck, boiled and salted	2.5	L	L
Duck, raw	2.5	L	L
Egg white, boiled	0.9	L	L
Egg white, raw	1.1	L	L
Egg yolk, boiled	0.5	L	L
Egg yolk, raw	0.6	L	L
Free-range, raw	2	L	L
Fried in sunflower oil	2	L	L
Fried in vegetable oil	2	L	L
Fried, without fat	1.8	L	L
Poached	1.8	L	L
Quail, raw	1.4	L	L

EGG DISHES

Omelette, cheese	5.3	L	L
Omelette, plain (two-egg)	4.2	L	L
Omelette, potato (two-egg)	5.3	L	L
Scrambled, with milk (two-egg)	4.2	L	L
Scrambled, without milk (two-egg)	3.5	L	L

MILK AND MILK SUBSTITUTES

Coffee creamer	0.1	L	L
Condensed milk, skim, sweetened	0.5	M	M
Condensed milk, whole, sweetened	0.5	M	M
Evaporated milk, reduced-fat	0.5	M	M
Evaporated milk, whole	0.5	M	H
Flavored milk	7.5	M	M
Goats' milk, pasteurized	5.2	L	L
Low-fat milk, pasteurized	5.2	L	L
Low-fat milk, UHT	5.2	L	L

Unless otherwise specified, figures are for one egg, chicken's eggs are medium-sized, and milk is cows' milk.

ENERGY cal	ENERGY J	FAT g	SATURATED FAT g	PROTEIN g	CARBO- HYDRATE g	FIBER g
79	328	5.4	1.5	7.6	0	0
72	298	4.8	1.4	7.1	0	0
139	575	2.7	11	10	Trace	0
122	510	2.2	9	11	Trace	0
14	60	0	0	3.5	0	0
14	59	0.1	0	3.5	0	0
54	224	4.9	1.4	2.5	0	0
62	259	5.6	1.6	3	0	0
86	358	1.7	7	7	Trace	0
120	499	9.4	2	8.8	0	0
107	447	2.4	8	8	Trace	0
87	363	1.8	6	8	Trace	0
75	309	5.3	1.5	6.7	0	0
60	252	1.2	4	5	Trace	0
399	1659	18.3	34	24	Trace	0
229	950	8.9	20	13	Trace	0
180	752	2.4	12	9	9	2.1
296	1230	13.9	27	13	1	0
160	664	3.3	12	14	Trace	0
16	68	1	1	0	2	0
40	171	0	0	2	9	0
50	211	2	0.9	1	8	0
18	77	1	0.2	1	2	0
23	94	1	0.9	1	1	0
146	614	3	1.9	8	23	0
88	369	5	3.4	5	6	0
67	285	2	1.5	5	7	0
67	283	2	1.6	5	7	0

MILK AND MILK SUBSTITUTES

	AVERAGE PORTION oz	GI	GL
Sheep's milk	5.2	L	L
Skim milk, dried	0.1	L	L
Skim milk, dried, with vegetable fat	0.1	L	L
Skim milk, pasteurized	5.2	L	L
Skim milk, sterilized	4.8	L	L
Skim milk, UHT	5.2	L	L
Soy milk	5.2	L	L
Soy milk, flavored	5.2	L	L
Whole milk, dried	0.1	L	L
Whole milk, pasteurized	5.2	L	L
Whole milk, sterilized	5.2	L	L
Whole milk, UHT	5.2	L	L

YOGURTS

	AVERAGE PORTION oz	GI	GL
Crème fraîche (see under cream)			
Fromage frais (see under cheese)			
Drinking yogurt	7	L	L
Probiotic yogurt drink, orange	3.5	M	M
Probiotic yogurt drink, plain	3.5	L	L
Yogurt, French set, fruit, low-fat	4.4	L	L
Yogurt, fruit	4.4	M	M
Yogurt, fruit, low-fat	4.4	L	L
Yogurt, fruit, virtually fat-free	4.4	L	L
Yogurt, Greek-style, fruit, whole milk	5.3	M	M
Yogurt, Greek-style, honey, whole milk	5.3	M	M
Yogurt, Greek-style, natural, whole milk	5.3	L	L
Yogurt, hazelnut, low-fat	4.4	L	L
Yogurt, long life, fruit, whole milk	4.4	M	M
Yogurt, natural, low-fat	4.4	L	L
Yogurt, natural, virtually fat-free	4.4	L	L
Yogurt, soy, fruit	4.4	M	M
Yogurt, twin pot, fruit, virtually fat-free	4.8	M	M
Yogurt, vanilla, low-fat	4.4	L	L

Unless otherwise specified, milk is cows' milk.

ENERGY cal	ENERGY J	FAT g	SATURATED FAT g	PROTEIN g	CARBO-HYDRATE g	FIBER g
139	578	8	5.5	8	7	0
10	44	0	0	1	2	0
15	61	1	0.5	1	1	0
48	204	1	0.1	5	7	0
44	188	1	0.1	5	7	0
47	200	1	0.1	5	7	0
47	193	2	0.4	4	1	Trace
58	245	2	0.3	4	5	Trace
15	62	1	0.5	1	1	0
96	402	6	3.5	5	7	0
96	404	6	3.5	5	7	0
96	402	6	3.5	5	7	0
124	526	Trace	Trace	6	26	Trace
67	279	0.9	0.6	1.5	13.4	1.3
68	284	1	0.7	1.7	13.1	1.4
103	435	1.4	1	4.3	19.5	0.3
133	564	3.8	2.5	4.9	21.4	0.3
97	412	1.4	0.9	5.1	17.1	0.3
75	318	0.5	0	5.9	12.5	0.3
205	857	12.6	8.4	7.2	16.8	Trace
221	927	12.5	8.4	7.7	21	Trace
198	824	15.3	10.2	8.4	7.2	Trace
111	469	1.9	0.8	5.5	19.1	0.3
125	529	4.3	0	3.9	19.1	0.3
69	294	1.3	0.9	5.9	9.3	Trace
67	286	0.3	0	6.6	10.3	Trace
92	388	2.3	0.3	2.9	16	0.4
55	236	0.1	0.1	4.5	9.7	0.7
114	484	1.1	0.8	4.8	22.6	Trace

FATS	AVERAGE PORTION oz	GI	GL
Butter			
Butter	0.7	L	L
Ghee	0.25	L	L
Margarine			
Hard block	0.5	L	L
Soft, animal and vegetable fat	0.25	L	L
Soft, polyunsaturated	0.25	L	L
Other fats			
Compound cooking fat	0.5	L	L
Compound cooking fat, polyunsaturated	0.5	L	L
Dripping, beef	0.5	L	L
Ghee, vegetable	0.25	L	L
Lard	0.5	L	L
Spreads			
Butter, spreadable (75–80% fat)	0.4	L	L
Butter, spreadable, light (60% fat)	0.4	L	L
Low-fat spread (26–39%)	0.25	L	L
Low-fat spread (26–39%) with olive oil	0.25	L	L
Low-fat spread (26–39%), polyunsaturated	0.25	L	L
Reduced-fat spread (41–62%)	0.25	L	L
Reduced-fat spread (41–62%) with olive oil	0.25	L	L
Reduced-fat spread (41–62%), polyunsaturated	0.25	L	L
Reduced-fat spread (62–75%)	0.25	L	L

OILS			
Canola oil	0.4	L	L
Corn oil	0.5	L	L
Flaxseed oil	0.5	L	L

ENERGY cal	ENERGY J	FAT g	SATURATED FAT g	PROTEIN g	CARBO-HYDRATE g	FIBER g
147	606	16	11	0	Trace	0
63	259	7	4.6	Trace	Trace	0
103	424	11.5	4	0	0	0
52	213	6	1.9	0	0	0
52	215	6	1.2	Trace	0	0
135	555	15	6.3	0	0	0
135	554	15	3.1	Trace	Trace	0
134	549	15	7.9	Trace	Trace	0
63	259	7	3.3	0	0	0
134	549	15	6	Trace	0	0
72	294	7.9	3.4	0	0.1	0
55	225	6	2.6	0.1	0.1	0
25	106	2.7	0.7	0	0.2	0
25	102	2.7	0.6	0	0	0
23	98	2.6	0.6	0	0.1	0
39	162	4.2	1.1	0	0.1	0
38	157	4.1	0.9	0	0.1	0
37	153	4.1	0.9	0	0	0
46	190	5.1	1.7	0	0	0
99	407	11	0.7	Trace	0	0
135	554	15	2.2	Trace	0	0
135	565	15	1.4	0	0	0

OILS	AVERAGE PORTION oz	GI	GL
Grapeseed oil	0.4	L	L
Hazelnut oil	0.1	L	L
Olive oil	0.4	L	L
Palm oil	0.4	L	L
Peanut oil	0.4	L	L
Safflower oil	0.4	L	L
Sesame oil	0.1	L	L
Soya oil	0.4	L	L
Sunflower oil	0.4	L	L
Vegetable oil	0.4	L	L
Walnut oil	0.4	L	L
Wheatgerm oil	0.4	L	L

ENERGY cal	ENERGY J	FAT g	SATURATED FAT g	PROTEIN g	CARBO-HYDRATE g	FIBER g
99	407	11	1.2	Trace	0	0
99	407	11	0.9	Trace	0	0
99	407	11	1.6	Trace	0	0
99	407	11	5.3	Trace	0	0
99	407	11	2.2	Trace	0	0
99	407	11	1.1	Trace	0	0
27	111	3	0.4	Trace	0	0
99	407	11	1 .7	Trace	0	0
99	407	11	1.3	Trace	0	0
99	407	11	1.1	Trace	0	0
99	407	11	1	Trace	0	0
99	407	11	2	Trace	0	0

SWEET SPREADS	AVERAGE PORTION oz	GI	GL
Chocolate spread	1.2	M	L
Fruit spread	0.6	M	L
Honey	0.6	M	L
Lemon curd	0.5	M	L

SAVORY SPREADS AND PÂTÉS			
Fish paste	0.4	L	L
Liver sausage	1.4	L	L
Mackerel pâté, smoked	1.4	L	L
Meat spread	0.4	L	L
Pâté, liver, tubed	1.4	L	L
Peanut butter, crunchy	0.9	L	L
Peanut butter, smooth	0.9	L	L
Tuna pâté	1.4	L	L
Vegetable pâté	2.8	L	L

JAMS AND MARMALADES			
Jam, diabetic	0.5	L	L
Jam, fruit with edible seeds	0.5	L	L
Jam, reduced-sugar	0.5	L	L
Jam, stone fruit	0.5	L	L
Marmalade	0.5	L	L
Marmalade, diabetic	0.5	L	L

Unless otherwise specified, spreads are made with polyunsaturated fats.

ENERGY cal	ENERGY J	FAT g	SATURATED FAT g	PROTEIN g	CARBO-HYDRATE g	FIBER g
201	841	13.2	2.8	1.2	20.8	0.4
19	83	Trace	Trace	0	5	0.1
49	209	0	0	0	13	0
42	180	1	0.2	0	9	0
17	71	1	0.5	2	0	0
90	377	7	2.1	5	2	0.3
147	608	14	2.5	5	1	Trace
19	80	1	0.6	2	0	Trace
114	472	10	3	5	0	Trace
152	628	13	2.4	6	2	1.5
156	645	13	2.9	6	3	1.4
94	393	7	3.1	7	0	Trace
138	574	11	6	6	5	2
26	109	0	0	0	9	0.1
39	167	0	0	0	10	0.1
18	78	Trace	Trace	0	5	0.1
39	167	0	0	0	10	0.1
39	167	0	0	0	10	0
26	109	0	0	0	9	0.1

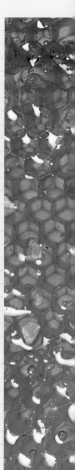

BREAKFAST CEREALS	AVERAGE PORTION oz	GI	GL
Bran, flakes	1	H	M
Bran, flakes with oat	1	M	M
Bran, raisin	1	H	M
Bran, strands	1.4	L	L
Bran, with oat and wheat	1.8	M	M
Corn flakes	1	H	H
Corn flakes, with nuts	1	H	M
Crunchy clusters	1.8	H	M
Crunchy clusters with fruit	1.8	H	M
Frosted flakes	1	H	H
Fruit and fiber breakfast cereal	1.4	H	H
Hoops, honey	1	H	H
Hoops, honey and nut	1	H	H
Malted flakes	1	M	M
Muesli	1.8	M	L
Muesli, crunchy with nuts	1.8	M	L
Muesli, Swiss-style	1.8	M	L
Muesli, with extra fruit	1.8	M	L
Muesli, with no added sugar	1.8	M	L
Multigrain flakes	1	M	M
Oat cereal with fruit and nuts	1.8	M	M
Oat cereal with tropical fruit	1.8	M	M
Oat clusters	1	M	M
Oat flakes	1	M	M
Oatmeal, instant, made with water	6.3	L	M
Oatmeal, made with water	5.6	L	L
Oatmeal, made with whole milk	5.6	L	L
Puffed rice	1	H	H
Puffed rice, chocolate	1	H	H
Puffed wheat	0.7	H	H
Wheat, shredded	1.6	M	M
Wheat, shredded, honey and nut	1.4	M	M
Wheat, shredded, mini	1.6	M	M
Wholewheat biscuits	0.7	M	M

All values are without any sugar added.

ENERGY cal	ENERGY J	FAT g	SATURATED FAT g	PROTEIN g	CARBO-HYDRATE g	FIBER g
95	406	1	0.1	3	21	3.9
105	435	2	0.2	3	20	3
96	405	1	0.1	3	18	3.9
104	444	1	0.2	6	19	9.8
163	691	2	0.3	5	34	8.9
108	461	Trace	0	2	26	0.3
119	507	1	0.2	2	27	0.2
200	844	5.8	2.1	3.6	35.5	2.2
139	580	5	1.7	4	20	1.3
113	482	Trace	0	2	28	0.2
147	614	2	1.2	2	28	2.2
111	465	1	0.2	2	23	2.1
112	474	1	0.3	2	23	1.5
186	773	1	0.1	3	23	1.3
184	770	3	0.7	6	33	3.2
225	946	10.3	2.3	4.2	31	2.2
182	770	3	0.4	5	36	3.2
186	789	3	0.4	5	37	3.2
183	776	4	0.8	5	34	3.8
111	465	Trace	Trace	5	22	0.7
213	888	8	3	5	31	2
217	905	7	4	4	34	3
116	490	3	0.8	3	20	2.7
107	456	1	0.2	3	22	3
671	2844	14	2.2	21	123	13
78	334	2	0.3	2	14	1.3
186	781	8	4.3	8	22	1.3
111	472	0.1	0.1	2	27	0.2
115	491	0.1	0.1	2	28	0.2
64	273	Trace	0	3	13	1.1
150	630	1	0.2	5	30	5.2
152	642	3	0.9	4	28	4.1
154	655	1	0.2	4	32	5
70	300	0.1	0.1	2	15	1.9

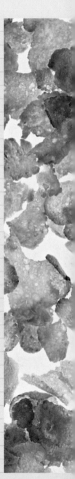

CRACKERS

	AVERAGE PORTION oz	GI	GL
Cheese, low sodium	0.5	M	M
Cheese, regular	0.5	M	M
Cheese, sandwich with peanut butter	0.5	M	M
Crackers, regular	0.5	M	M
Crackers, regular, low salt	0.5	M	M
Crackers, sandwich, with cheese	0.5	M	M
Crackers, sandwich, with peanut butter	0.5	M	M
Milk crackers	0.8	M	M
Nabisco wheat thins	1	M	M
Oat crackers	0.7	L	L
Rye, sandwich with cheese	0.5	M	M
Rye, wafers, plain	0.9	M	M
Rye, wafers, seasoned	0.8	M	M
Saltines, fat-free, low sodium	0.5	M	M
Saltines, low salt	0.5	M	M
Saltines, regular	0.5	M	M
Saltines, unsalted tops	0.5	M	M
Wheat, low salt	0.5	M	M
Wheat, regular	0.5	M	M
Wheat, sandwich, with cheese	0.5	M	M
Wheat, sandwich, with peanut butter	0.5	M	M
Whole-wheat	0.5	M	M
Whole-wheat, low salt	0.5	M	M

CRISPBREADS

Breadsticks	0.3	M	M
Crispbakes	0.6	H	H
Crispbread, rye	1.3	M	M
Matzo, egg	0.5	M	M
Matzo, egg and onion	0.5	M	M
Matzo, plain	0.5	M	M
Matzo, whole-wheat	0.5	M	M
Melba toast, plain	0.5	M	M

Unless otherwise specified, a helping is two biscuits.

ENERGY cal	ENERGY J	FAT g	SATURATED FAT g	PROTEIN g	CARBO- HYDRATE g	FIBER g
75	316	4	1.4	2	9	0.4
75	316	4	1.4	2	9	0.4
72	303	3	0.8	2	9	0.4
75	315	4	0.6	1	9	0.2
75	315	4	0.6	1	9	0.2
72	299	3	0.9	1	9	0.3
73	306	4	0.8	2	9	0.4
100	419	3	0.6	2	15	0.4
136	570	6	0.9	2	20	0.9
91	381	4	1.1	1.9	12.6	1.8
67	282	3	0.8	1	9	0.5
84	349	0	0	2	20	5.7
84	351	2	0.3	2	16	4.6
59	247	0	0	2	12	0.4
65	272	2	0.4	1	11	0.4
65	272	2	0.4	1	11	0.4
65	272	2	0.4	1	11	0.4
71	297	3	0.8	1	10	0.7
71	297	3	0.8	1	10	0.7
75	312	4	0.6	1	9	0.5
74	311	4	0.7	2	8	0.7
66	278	3	0.5	1	10	1.6
66	278	3	0.5	1	10	1.6
39	165	0.8	0.6	1.1	7.3	0.2
60	250	Trace	Trace	2	12	0.6
105	448	0.5	0.1	3.2	23.5	5.3
59	245	0	0.1	2	12	0.4
59	245	1	0.1	2	12	0.8
59	248	0	0	2	13	0.4
53	220	0	0	2	12	1.8
58	245	0	0.1	2	11	0.9

CRISPBREADS	AVERAGE PORTION oz	GI	GL
Melba toast, plain, without salt	0.5	M	M
Melba toast, rye	0.5	M	M
Melba toast, wheat	0.5	M	M
Rice cakes	0.6	H	H

COOKIES			
Animal crackers	0.5	H	M
Archway, apple-filled oatmeal	0.9	H	M
Archway, coconut macaroon	0.8	H	M
Archway, date-filled oatmeal	0.9	M	M
Archway, gourmet oatmeal pecan	1	M	M
Archway, iced oatmeal	1	H	M
Archway, oatmeal	0.9	M	M
Archway, oatmeal raisin	0.9	M	M
Chocolate chip	1	H	M
Chocolate-coated shortcake	0.8	H	M
Chocolate grahams	1	H	M
Chocolate sandwich, with creme filling, chocolate-coated	0.7	H	M
Chocolate wafers	0.5	H	M
Coconut macaroons, homemade	0.8	H	M
Fig bars	0.6	H	M
Ginger nuts	0.7	H	M
Granola bars, with fruit and/or nuts	0.9	M	M
Granola bars, with fruit and/or nuts and chocolate	0.9	M	M
Ice cream sandwich wafers, plain not filled	0.3	H	H
Marshmallows, chocolate-coated	0.9	H	H
Oatmeal, with raisins, homemade	1.1	L	M
Oatmeal, without raisins, homemade	1.1	L	L
Oatmeal, regular, store bought	0.8	L	L
Oatmeal, soft-type, store bought	1.1	L	L

Unless otherwise specified, a helping is two biscuits.

ENERGY cal	ENERGY J	FAT g	SATURATED FAT g	PROTEIN g	CARBO-HYDRATE g	FIBER g
58	245	0	0.1	2	11	0.9
58	244	1	0.1	2	12	1.2
56	235	0	0.1	2	11	1.1
56	234	Trace	Trace	2	12	0.8
67	80	2	0.5	1	11	0.2
98	412	3	0.7	1	16	0.5
106	444	6	5.4	1	12	0.5
99	413	3	0.7	1	17	0.7
134	559	7	2.4	2	16	0.8
123	514	5	1.5	1	18	0.6
106	444	4	0.9	2	17	0.7
107	446	4	0.8	1	17	0.8
123	517	6	2.7	1.5	17	0.5
132	551	7.1	3.9	1.7	16.3	0.6
136	567	6	3.7	2	19	0.9
99	415	5.6	3.2	1	11.8	0.4
52	217	2	0.5	1	9	0.4
97	406	3	2.7	1	17	0.4
65	276	1.9	0.9	0.7	12	0.6
89	373	3.1	1.5	1	15.1	0.3
99	419	3	1.1	1.6	17.6	1
122	514	5.1	2.4	1.7	18.5	0.8
37	156	0.3	0.1	1	8	0.2
109	458	4	1.2	1	18	0.5
130	546	5	1	2	21	0.8
134	561	5	1.1	2	20	0.8
112	471	5	1.1	2	17	0.7
123	513	4	1.1	2	20	0.8

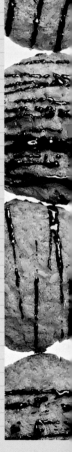

SAVORY SNACKS	AVERAGE PORTION oz	GI	GL
Bombay mix	1	M	M
Breadsticks	0.9	M	M
Cheese and potato puffs	0.9	H	M
Cheese balls	1.2	H	M
Cheese straws/twists	0.8	M	M
Chips, corn-based, plain	1	H	M
Corn snacks	0.9	H	M
Oriental mix	1.8	H	M
Popcorn, candied	2.6	H	H
Popcorn, salted	2.6	L	L
Pork scratchings	0.8	M	M
Potato and corn sticks	0.7	H	M
Potato and corn, waffle-shaped snacks	1.8	H	M
Potato chips	1	H	M
Potato chips, crinkle cut	1.4	H	M
Potato chips, fried in sunflower oil	1	H	M
Potato chips, jacket	1.4	M	M
Potato chips, low-fat	1	H	M
Potato chips, square	0.8	H	M
Potato chips, thick, crinkle cut	1.4	H	M
Potato chips, thick cut	1.4	H	M
Potato rings	1	H	M
Pretzels	1	H	M
Taco chips	0.9	H	M
Tortilla chips, nacho-flavor	1	H	M
Tortilla chips, nacho-flavor, light	1	H	M
Tortilla chips, nacho-flavor, made with enriched masa flour	1	H	M
Tortilla chips, plain	1	H	M
Tortilla chips, ranch-flavor	1	H	M
Tortilla chips, taco-flavor	1	H	M
Trail mix	0.8	M	M
Vegetable chips	1.4	H	M

ENERGY cal	ENERGY J	FAT g	SATURATED FAT g	PROTEIN g	CARBO-HYDRATE g	FIBER g
151	630	10	1.2	6	11	1.9
108	464	4	1.6	4	20	0.8
140	585	9	3.2	2	15	0.3
148	621	8	1.8	2	19	0.8
122	512	7.3	4.2	3.4	11.6	0.6
151	631	9	1.3	2	16	1.4
147	616	8.5	0.8	1.7	17	0.4
273	1142	20	3	10	17	0.3
360	1514	14	1.5	2	58	1
445	1851	32	3.2	5	37	1
133	554	10	3.6	11	0	0.1
88	368	4	1.3	1	11	0.6
241	1009	12	2.8	2	32	1.3
156	650	9.5	2.5	1.3	17.2	0.7
219	913	14	5.8	2	22	2.3
150	629	8.9	0.9	1.8	16.7	1.4
204	851	13	5.3	3	21	1.9
137	577	6	2.8	2	19	1.8
108	454	5	2.2	2	14	1.1
203	848	12	5	2	22	1.6
200	836	11	4.6	3	23	1.6
144	605	6.7	0.6	1.1	21.2	0.5
114	479	1	0.2	3	24	0.8
124	521	6	1.6	1	17	1.8
139	584	7	1.4	2	17	1.5
125	521	4	0.8	2	20	1.3
139	584	7	1.4	2	17	1.5
140	587	7	1.4	2	18	1.8
137	574	7	1.3	2	18	1.1
134	562	7	1.3	2	18	1.5
108	451	7	1.3	2	9	1.1
192	804	13.9	1.6	1.9	15.8	5

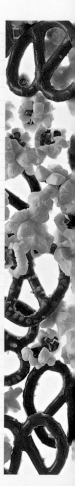

FLOUR	AVERAGE PORTION oz	GI	GL
Corn starch	1	H	M
Garbanzo (gram/chickpea)	3.5	H	H
Millet	3.5	L	H
Rice	3.5	H	H
Rye, whole	0.7	M	H
Wheat, white, bread	3.5	H	H
Wheat, white, all-purpose	3.5	H	H
Wheat, white, self-rising	3.5	H	H
Wheat, whole-wheat	3.5	M	H

GRAVY AND STOCK			
Fish stock, homemade	8.2	L	L
Gravy, chicken, canned	8.4	L	L
Gravy, au jus, canned	8.4	L	L
Gravy, beef, canned	8.2	L	L
Gravy, instant granules	0.2	L	L
Gravy, turkey, canned	8.4	L	L
Stock cubes, beef/chicken	0.25	L	L
Stock cubes, vegetable	0.25	L	L

MISCELLANEOUS			
Artichoke hearts, bottled in oil, drained	1.8	L	L
Baking soda	0.2	L	L
Bran, wheat	0.25	M	L
Capers in brine, drained	0.3	L	L
Chocolate chips, dark	3.5	H	H
Chocolate chips, milk	3.5	H	H
Chocolate chips, white	3.5	H	H
Coconut, creamed block	0.8	L	L
Coconut, desiccated	0.9	L	L
Coconut milk	3.5	L	L
Coconut milk, light	3.5	L	L

Unless otherwise specified, all gravies and stocks do not contain flour.

ENERGY cal	ENERGY J	FAT g	SATURATED FAT g	PROTEIN g	CARBO- HYDRATE g	FIBER g
106	452	0	0	0	28	0
313	1328	5.4	0.5	19.7	49.6	10.7
354	1481	1.7	0.7	5.8	75.4	8.5
366	1531	0.8	0.1	6.4	80.1	2
67	286	1	0.1	2	15	2.3
341	1451	1	0.2	12	75	3.1
341	1450	1	0.2	9	78	3.1
330	1407	1	0.2	9	76	3.1
310	1318	2	0.3	13	64	9
40	165	2	0.5	5	0	0
188	788	14	3.4	5	13	1
38	159	0	0.2	3	6	0
123	517	5	2.7	9	11	0.9
23	96	2	Trace	0	2	Trace
121	507	5	1 .5	6	12	1
17	69	1	Trace	1	1	0
18	74	1	Trace	1	1	Trace
63	265	4.2	0.6	1.6	5.1	2.5
0	0	0	0	0	0	0
14	61	1	0.1	1	2	2.5
4	15	0.1	0	0.2	0.5	0.3
496	2075	30	17.7	4.1	55.8	1.3
502	2101	27.6	14.4	5.6	61.6	0.8
531	2225	32.1	28.6	7.1	57.1	0
167	690	17	14.8	2	2	2
169	698	17	15	2	2	3.8
153	642	15	13.3	1.4	3.4	0.1
72	301	7	6.2	0.7	1.6	0.2

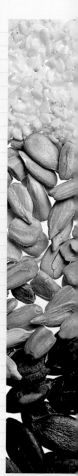

MISCELLANEOUS	AVERAGE PORTION oz	GI	GL
Gelatine	0.1	L	L
Marzipan, store bought	0.8	H	H
Olives, green, stuffed	1.4	L	L
Olives, in brine, pitted	0.6	L	L
Olives, mixed	1.4	L	L
Olives, mixed with feta	1.8	L	L
Pancake mix, plain (with buttermilk)	3.5	H	H
Thai green curry paste	0.5	L	L
Thai red curry paste	0.5	L	L
Tomato purée	0.5	L	L
Tomatoes, sundried, bottled in oil	0.4	L	L
Vegetable purée	0.7	L	L
Vinegar	0.5	L	L
Vinegar, cider	0.5	L	L
Wheatgerm	0.2	M	L
Yeast, bakers', compressed	0.2	L	L
Yeast, dried	0.2	L	L

SUGARS, SYRUPS AND TREACLE			
Sugar, brown	0.7	M	M
Sugar, Demerara	0.7	M	M
Sugar, icing	0.7	M	M
Sugar, white	0.7	M	M
Syrup, golden	1.9	M	M
Syrup, maple	0.7	M	M
Treacle, black	1.8	M	M

NUTS AND SEEDS			
Almonds, toasted	0.5	L	L
Brazil nuts	0.4	L	L
Caraway seeds	0.4	L	L
Cashew nuts, plain	0.4	L	L

ENERGY cal	ENERGY J	FAT g	SATURATED FAT g	PROTEIN g	CARBO-HYDRATE g	FIBER g
10	43	0	0	3	0	0
101	426	3	0.3	1	17	0.5
52	219	5	0.7	0.4	1.5	1.2
19	76	2	0.3	0	Trace	0.5
45	188	3.8	0.5	0.4	2.4	1.2
78	326	7.5	0.7	2.2	0.4	0.3
376	1573	5	1	10	71	2.7
17	71	1.2	0.5	0.3	1.3	0.5
25	103	2.1	0.1	0.1	1.4	0.2
10	43	0	0	0.7	1.9	0.5
50	204	5	0.7	0	1	0.5
14	51	1	0	1	1	0.6
3	13	0	0	0	0	0
2	9	0	0	0	1	0
18	75	0	0.1	1	2	0.8
3	11	0	0	1	0	Trace
8	36	0	0	2	0	Trace
72	309	0	0	0	20	0
79	336	0	0	0	21	0
79	336	0	0	Trace	21	0
79	336	0	0	Trace	21	0
164	698	0	0	0	43	0
52	219	0	0	0	13.4	0
129	548	0	0	1	34	Trace
81	334	7	0.6	3	1	1
68	281	7	1.6	1	0	0.4
40	169	1.5	0.1	2	5	3.8
57	237	5	1	2	2	0.3

NUTS AND SEEDS

	AVERAGE PORTION oz	GI	GL
Chestnuts	50	L	L
Chia seeds	0.4	L	L
Coconut, fresh	0.9	L	L
Flax seeds	0.4	L	L
Hazelnuts	0.4	L	L
Hemp seeds	0.4	L	L
Macadamia nuts, salted	0.4	L	L
Peanuts, dry roasted	1.4	L	L
Peanuts, plain	0.5	L	L
Pecan nuts	2	L	L
Pine nuts	0.2	L	L
Pistachio nuts, roasted and salted	0.4	L	L
Poppy seeds	0.4	L	L
Pumpkin seeds	0.6	L	L
Sesame seeds	0.5	L	L
Sunflower seeds	0.6	L	L
Walnuts	0.7	L	L

SOUP

	AVERAGE PORTION oz	GI	GL
Beef noodle	8.6	M	M
Black bean	8.7	L	M
Carrot and cilantro	10.6	M	M
Chicken corn chowder, chunky	8.5	M	M
Chicken gumbo	8.6	M	M
Chicken noodle, chunky	8.6	M	M
Crab	8.6	H	H
Cream of tomato	10.6	H	H
Leek and potato	10.6	M	H
Lentil	10.6	M	H
Mushroom barley	8.6	L	M
Split pea	10.6	M	M
Turkey noodle	8.6	M	M
Vegetable	8.5	L	L

ENERGY cal	ENERGY J	FAT g	SATURATED FAT g	PROTEIN g	CARBO- HYDRATE g	FIBER g
85	360	1	0.3	1	18	2
51	213	3.1	0.3	1.6	4.4	3.8
98	405	10	8.7	1	1	2
56	234	4.2	0.4	1.8	2.9	2.7
65	269	6	0.5	1	1	0.7
60	250	4.7	0.3	3.7	0.7	0.2
75	308	8	1.1	1	0	0.5
236	976	20	3.6	10	4	2.6
73	304	6	1.1	3	2	0.8
413	1706	42	3.4	6	3	2.8
34	142	3	0.2	1	0	0.1
60	249	6	0.7	2	1	0.6
57	237	4.5	0.5	1.8	2.4	1
91	378	7	1.1	4	2	0.8
72	296	7	1	2	0	0.9
96	400	8	0.8	3	3	1
138	567	14	1.1	3	1	0.7
83	346	3	1.1	5	9	0.7
116	487	2	0.4	6	20	4.4
130	544	7.8	3	1.7	14.1	4.5
238	994	15	4.2	7	18	2.2
56	234	1	0.3	3	8	2
114	479	3	0.8	8	14	2
76	317	2	0.4	5	10	0.7
186	774	10.2	1.5	2.7	21.9	1.5
168	705	8.4	4.7	5.1	18.6	2.4
117	492	0.6	0	9.3	19.5	3.6
73	307	2	0.4	2	12	0.7
154	644	2.8	1.3	8.3	25.4	4.8
68	285	2	0.6	4	9	0.7
72	304	2	0.3	2	12	0.5

TABLE SAUCES	AVERAGE PORTION oz	GI	GL
Applesauce, homemade	0.7	M	L
Applesauce, sweetened, canned	1	M	M
Applesauce, unsweetened, canned	1.3	M	L
Balsamic vinegar	0.5	L	L
Chili sauce	0.8	M	L
Cranberry sauce, canned, sweetened	2	M	L
Horseradish sauce	0.7	M	L
Mint sauce	0.4	M	L
Mustard, powder, made up	0.3	L	L
Mustard, smooth	0.1	L	L
Mustard, wholegrain	0.5	L	L
Soy sauce, dark, thick	0.2	M	L
Soy sauce, light, thin	0.2	M	L
Tartar sauce	1	M	L
Tomato ketchup	0.7	M	L
Worcestershire sauce	0.4	L	L

DRESSINGS AND MAYONNAISE			
Blue and roquefort cheese dressing	0.5	M	M
Blue cheese dressing	0.8	M	M
Caesar dressing	0.5	M	M
"Fat-free" dressing	0.5	L	L
French dressing	0.5	L	L
French dressing, diet, low-fat	0.6	L	L
Honey mustard dressing	0.5	M	M
Italian dressing, diet	0.5	L	L
Italian dressing	0.5	L	L
Kraft Free fat-free Italian dressing	0.5	L	L
Kraft Free fat-free ranch dressing	0.5	L	L
Kraft Light Done Right! Italian dressing	0.5	L	L
Kraft Light Done Right! ranch dressing	0.5	L	L
Kraft fat-free mayonnaise dressing	0.6	L	L

ENERGY cal	ENERGY J	FAT g	SATURATED FAT g	PROTEIN g	CARBO-HYDRATE g	FIBER g
13	55	0	0	0	3	0.2
23	95	0	0	0	6	0.4
15	63	0	0	0	4	0.4
15	63	0	0	0	4	0
20	84	Trace	Trace	0	4	0.3
86	360	0	0	0	22	0.6
31	128	2	0.2	1	4	0.5
10	43	Trace	Trace	0	2	0.2
18	75	1	0.1	1	0	0
3	12	0	0	0	0	0
20	82	1	0.1	1	5	Trace
3	13	0	0	0	6	0.2
3	13	Trace	Trace	0	1	0.7
90	372	7	0.5	0	0	0.2
23	98	Trace	Trace	0	1	0.7
6	28	0	0	0.1	1.6	0
76	316	8	1.5	1	1	0
114	472	12	6.2	1	2	0
65	271	6.9	1.3	0.2	0.5	0
10	42	0	0	0	2	0
64	270	6	1.4	0	3	0
21	90	1	0.1	0	3	0
49	205	2.6	0.3	0.1	6.7	0.1
16	66	1	0.2	0	1	0
70	293	7	1	0	2	0
9	39	0	0.1	0	2	0.1
21	87	0	0	0	5	0.1
26	107	2	0.2	0	1	0.2
38	161	3	0.3	0	2	0.1
11	47	0	0.1	0	2	0.3

DRESSINGS AND MAYONNAISE	AVERAGE PORTION oz	GI	GL
Kraft light mayonnaise	0.5	L	L
Kraft Miracle Whip Free nonfat dressing	0.6	L	L
Kraft Miracle Whip light dressing	0.6	L	L
Kraft ranch dressing	0.5	M	M
Kraft zesty Italian dressing	0.5	L	L
Low-fat dressing	0.5	L	L
Mayonnaise, store bought	1	L	L
Mayonnaise, homemade, made with lemon juice	1	L	L
Mayonnaise, homemade, made with vinegar	1	L	L
Mayonnaise, reduced-calorie	1	L	L
Mayonnaise, imitation, milk cream	0.5	L	L
Mayonnaise, imitation, soybean	0.5	L	L
Mayonnaise, imitation, soybean without cholesterol	0.5	L	L
Mayonnaise, soybean and safflower oil	0.5	L	L
Mayonnaise, soybean oil	0.5	L	L
Oil and lemon dressing	0.5	L	L
Ranch salad dressing	0.5	M	M
Russian dressing, low calorie	0.6	L	L
Sesame seed dressing	0.5	L	L
Thousand island dressing	1	L	L
Thousand island, dressing reduced-calorie	1	L	L
Yogurt-based dressing	1	L	L

WHITE SAUCES

	AVERAGE PORTION oz	GI	GL
Cheese sauce, made with low-fat milk	2.2	M	M
Cheese sauce, made with whole milk	2.2	M	M
Hollandaise, store bought	1	M	M
Hollandaise, homemade	1	M	M
Onion sauce, made with low-fat milk	2.2	M	M

ENERGY cal	ENERGY J	FAT g	SATURATED FAT g	PROTEIN g	CARBO- HYDRATE g	FIBER g
50	210	5	0.8	0	1	0
13	56	0	0.1	0	2	0.3
37	155	3	0.5	0	2	0
76	320	8	1.2	0	1	0
53	220	5	0.6	0	1	0.1
11	45	1	0.1	0	1	Trace
206	847	22.4	1.7	0.3	0.7	0
237	974	26	3.8	1	0	Trace
217	894	24	3.5	1	0	0
86	356	8	1.1	0	2	0
14	61	1	0.4	0	2	0
35	145	3	0.5	0	2	0
67	282	7	1	0	2	0
100	420	11	1.2	0	0	0
100	420	11	1.7	0	0	0
97	399	11	1.1	0	0	Trace
74	309	7.7	1.4	0.2	1	0.1
23	95	1	0.1	0	4	0
66	278	7	0.9	0	1	0.2
97	401	9	0.9	0	4	0.1
59	243	5	0.5	0	4	Trace
88	363	8	0.8	1	3	Trace
112	465	8	3.9	4	6	0.1
122	508	8	4.8	4	6	0.1
136	570	14.2	8.3	1.5	0.6	0
215	900	23.1	13.8	1.5	0.3	0
53	224	3	1.1	2	5	0.2

	AVERAGE PORTION oz	GI	GL
WHITE SAUCES			
Onion sauce, made with whole milk	2.2	M	M
White sauce, savory, made with low-fat milk	2.2	M	M
White sauce, savory, made with whole milk	2.2	M	M
White sauce, sweet, made with low-fat milk	2.2	M	M
White sauce, sweet, made with whole milk	2.2	M	M
CHUTNEYS			
Chutney, apple, homemade	1.2	M	M
Chutney, mango, sweet	1.2	M	M
Chutney, tomato	1.2	M	M
DIPS			
Dips, sour-cream-based	1	L	L
Guacamole	1.6	L	L
Hummus	1	L	L
Salsa	1	L	L
Taramasalata	1.6	L	L
Tzatziki	1.6	L	L
PICKLES			
Gherkins, pickled	0.8	L	L
Onions, pickled	1	L	L
Pickle, chilli, oily	0.5	L	L
Pickle, lime, oily	0.5	L	L
Pickle, mango, oily	0.5	L	L
Pickle, mixed vegetables	0.5	L	L
Pickle, sweet	0.5	L	L

ENERGY cal	ENERGY J	FAT g	SATURATED FAT g	PROTEIN g	CARBO- HYDRATE g	FIBER g
61	257	4	1.7	2	5	0.2
79	334	5	1.8	3	7	0.1
93	387	6	2.7	3	7	0.1
93	393	4	1.7	2	12	0.1
105	441	6	2.5	2	12	0.1
66	283	Trace	Trace	0	17	0.4
62	266	Trace	Trace	0	16	0.3
42	179	Trace	Trace	0	10	0.4
108	445	11	3.7	1	1	Trace
58	239	6	1.2	1	1	1.1
56	234	4	0.5	2	3	0.7
20	86	1.1	0	0.3	2.5	0.4
227	935	24	1.8	1	2	Trace
30	124	2	1.3	2	1	0.1
4	15	Trace	Trace	0	1	0.3
7	30	Trace	Trace	0	1	0.4
41	168	4	Trace	0	1	0.2
27	111	2	Trace	0	1	0.2
27	110	2	Trace	0	1	0.2
3	14	0	0	0	1	0.2
21	91	0	Trace	0	5	0.2

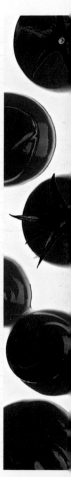

COOKING SAUCES

	AVERAGE PORTION oz	GI	GL
Barbecue sauce	0.8	M	L
Black bean sauce	0.7	M	L
Bolognese sauce, fresh	3.5	L	M
Carbonara sauce, fresh	3.5	L	M
Chili sauce	0.8	M	L
Chinese stir fry sauce	5	M	L
Curry sauce, canned	5.3	M	L
Curry sauce with tomato and onion	5.3	M	M
Fish sauce	0.4	L	L
Four cheese sauce, fresh	3.5	M	M
Hoisin sauce	0.6	M	L
Korma cook-in sauce	5	M	M
Oyster sauce	0.5	L	L
Pesto, green	3.5	L	M
Pesto, red	3.5	L	M
Plum sauce	0.7	M	L
Sofrito sauce	0.5	L	M
Soy sauce	0.2	L	L
Spaghetti marinara sauce, ready-to-serve	4.4	L	M
Spaghetti sauce, meatless, canned	9.6	L	M
Sweet and sour cook-in sauce	5	L	M
Tabasco	0.2	L	L
Teriyaki sauce	0.7	M	L
Tomato sauce, fresh	3.5	L	M
Tomato sauce with vegetables, fresh	3.5	L	M
White milk/cream-based cook-in sauce	5	M	M

CUSTARDS

Crème caramel	3.2	L	L
Crème patissiere	5.3	L	L
Custard, made with low-fat milk	5.3	L	L
Custard, made with whole milk	4.2	L	L

ENERGY cal	ENERGY J	FAT g	SATURATED FAT g	PROTEIN g	CARBO- HYDRATE g	FIBER g
23	99	0	0	0	6	0.1
19	79	0	0	1	2	0.4
44	182	1.3	0.2	1.5	6.9	1.3
151	632	13	7.7	4.9	3.8	0.4
20	84	Trace	Trace	0	4	0.3
129	539	1.8	0.2	2	27.9	1.1
117	486	8	0.4	2	11	Trace
297	1229	29	3	3	9	1.7
4	15	0	0	0.5	0.4	0
164	685	12.3	7.3	5.1	8.7	0.9
35	147	1	0.1	1	7	0.4
186	781	13.3	6.1	2.4	15.3	2.1
12	51	0	Trace	1	3	Trace
412	1725	42.5	6.5	3.7	3.9	1.1
307	1284	30.6	4.7	5	3	1
35	146	0	0	0	8	0.1
36	149	3	0	2	1	0.3
3	13	0	0	0	0	0
71	298	3	0.4	2	10	2
129	541	2	0.4	3	23	3
131	550	1.4	0.2	0.7	30.9	1.3
1	2	0	0	0	0	0
15	63	0	0	1	3	0
33	140	0.3	0.1	1.4	6.7	1.8
46	192	2.1	0.3	1.4	5.7	2.4
147	614	12	2.4	2.2	7.8	2.7
98	416	1	Trace	3	19	Trace
255	1077	9	4.1	10	37	0.3
141	605	3	1.8	6	25	Trace
140	594	5	3.4	4	20	Trace

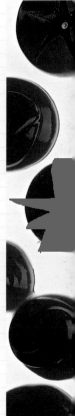

PASTRY	AVERAGE PORTION oz	GI	GL
Cheese	3.5	H	H
Choux	3.5	H	H
Filo, cooked	3.5	H	H
Filo, uncooked	3.5	H	H
Flaky, cooked	3.5	H	H
Flaky, uncooked	3.5	H	H
Pie	3.5	H	H
Puff, cooked	1.4	H	H
Puff, uncooked	1.4	H	H
Whole-wheat	3.5	H	H

SWEET PASTRIES			
Asian pastries	1.4	M	H
Chinese flaky pastries	1.4	H	H
Croissants, plain	2	H	M
Danish pastry, cheese	2.5	H	H
Danish pastry, cinnamon	1.9	H	H
Danish pastry, fruit	1.9	H	H
Danish pastry, nut	1.9	H	H
Danish pastry, raspberry	2.5	H	H
Greek pastries	3.5	H	H

PASTRY DISHES			
Beef pie, individual	5.3	H	L
Chicken and mushroom pie	3.5	H	H
Chicken pie, individual, baked	4.6	H	H
Quiche, broccoli	5	H	H
Quiche, broccoli, whole-wheat	5	H	H
Quiche, cauliflower and cheese	5	H	H
Quiche, cauliflower and cheese, whole-wheat	5	H	H
Quiche, cheese and egg	5	H	H

Unless otherwise specified, all pastry dishes are homemade.

ENERGY cal	ENERGY J	FAT g	SATURATED FAT g	PROTEIN g	CARBO-HYDRATE g	FIBER g
500	2083	34	15.3	13	37	1.5
325	1355	20	15	9	30	1.2
363	1544	3.8	0.4	10	77.1	2.2
278	1180	2.9	0.3	7.6	58.9	1.7
547	2281	37.9	14.1	6.9	47.5	2.2
453	1889	31.4	11.7	5.7	39.4	1.8
521	2174	32	11.7	7	54	2.2
486	2027	33.2	15.9	6.7	42.8	1.1
384	1600	26.2	12.6	5.3	33.7	0.9
499	2080	33	11.8	9	45	6.3
215	897	16	8	3	17	0.8
157	659	7	4	2	24	0.8
224	938	12	5.9	5	26	1
266	1111	16	4.8	6	26	0.7
214	894	12	3	4	24	0.7
197	823	10	2.6	3	25	1
228	953	13	3.1	4	24	1.1
263	1102	13	2	4	34	1.3
456	1909	25.1	9.7	6.7	54.1	1.6
438	1830	26.6	11.9	13.8	38.3	2
200	836	10	4.5	13	14	0.6
374	1563	21	9.1	12	32	1
349	1455	21	8.3	12	30	1.7
337	1408	21	8.3	13	25	3.8
277	1156	18	7.1	7	24	1.5
269	1121	18	7.1	8	20	3.1
440	1834	31	14.4	18	24	0.8

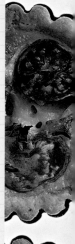
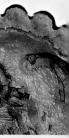

PASTRY DISHES	AVERAGE PORTION oz	GI	GL
Quiche, cheese and egg, whole-wheat	5	H	H
Quiche, cheese and mushroom	5	H	H
Quiche, cheese and mushroom, wholewheat	5	H	H
Quiche, cheese, onion and potato	5	H	H
Quiche, cheese, onion and potato, wholewheat	5	H	H
Quiche, fish, store bought	5	H	H
Quiche, meat, store bought	5	H	
Quiche, mushroom	5	H	H
Quiche, mushroom, whole-wheat	5	H	H
Quiche, spinach	5	H	H
Quiche, spinach, whole-wheat	5	H	H
Quiche, vegetable, store bought	5	H	H
Quiche, vegetable, whole-wheat	5	H	H

TOASTER PASTRIES			
Kellogg's Pop-Tarts, blueberry	1.8	M	H
Kellogg's Pop-Tarts, brown sugar cinnamon	1.8	M	H
Kellogg's Pop-Tarts, frosted blueberry	1.8	M	H
Kellogg's Pop-Tarts, frosted brown sugar cinnamon	1.8	M	H
Kellogg's Pop-Tarts, frosted cherry	1.8	M	H
Kellogg's Pop-Tarts, frosted chocolate fudge	1.8	M	H
Kellogg's Pop-Tarts, frosted raspberry	1.8	M	H
Kellogg's Pop-Tarts, frosted strawberry	1.8	M	H
Kellogg's Pop-Tarts, strawberry	1.8	M	H

Unless otherwise specified, all pastry dishes are homemade.

ENERGY cal	ENERGY J	FAT g	SATURATED FAT g	PROTEIN g	CARBO- HYDRATE g	FIBER g
431	1796	31	14.6	18	20	2.7
396	1655	26	10.8	15	26	1.3
388	1616	27	10.8	16	22	3.1
480	2005	33	16	18	28	1.4
472	1966	34	16.1	19	25	3.1
407	1702	25.9	10.9	13.7	31.6	1.5
474	1985	29.7	11.9	13.6	40.7	1.8
398	1659	27	12.2	14	26	1.3
388	1618	28	12.2	15	21	3.1
287	1203	18	5.6	14	18	2
281	1176	18	5.6	15	16	3.2
405	1695	27.6	11.5	11.3	29.7	2.5
286	1197	18	6	8	24	3.9
212	888	7	1.1	2	36	0.6
219	916	9	1	3	32	0.8
203	851	5	1	2	37	0.6
211	883	7	1.1	2	34	0.6
204	855	5	1	2	37	0.5
201	842	5	1	3	37	0.6
205	860	6	1	2	37	0.5
203	849	5	1.4	2	38	0.5
205	857	5	1.5	2	37	0.6

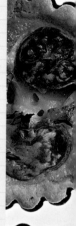
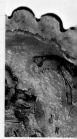

MILK-BASED PUDDINGS AND DESSERTS	AVERAGE PORTION oz	GI	GL
Milk pudding, made with low-fat milk	7	H	H
Milk pudding, made with whole milk	7	H	H
Rice desserts, individual, with fruit	4.8	H	H
Rice pudding, canned	7	H	H
Tiramisu	3.5	H	H
Trifle, chocolate	4	H	H
Trifle, fruit	4	H	H

CHEESECAKES			
Chocolate	4.2	H	H
Frozen	3.2	H	H
Fruit, individual	3.2	H	H
Fruit, large	4.2	H	H

OTHER DESSERTS			
Crumble, fruit	6	H	H
Jell-o, made with water	4	H	H
Plum pudding	3.5	H	H
Profiteroles with chocolate sauce	5.5	H	H
Sponge pudding	3.5	H	H
Sticky toffee pudding	3.5	H	H
Strudel, fruit	4	H	H

MOUSSE			
Chocolate, individual	2	H	H
Chocolate	2	H	H
Fruit	2	H	H

ENERGY cal	ENERGY J	FAT g	SATURATED FAT g	PROTEIN g	CARBO-HYDRATE g	FIBER g
214	914	4	2.2	8	40	0.2
258	1086	9	5.4	8	40	0.2
153	648	3	2	4	29	0.4
178	748	3	3.2	7	28	0.4
275	1149	18.2	10.5	4.8	24.4	0.9
233	971	17	10.7	5	15	1.4
161	672	10	6.3	3	15	2.4
415	1731	28	14.4	6	37	0.8
218	915	10	5	5	30	0.8
238	1000	11	6.8	5	31	0.9
353	1477	19	11.8	5	42	1
373	1571	14	6.7	4	61	2.2
70	299	0	0	1	17	0
291	1227	10	4.5	5	50	1.3
535	2226	40	21.7	9	38	1.1
343	1437	16.8	3.7	5.7	45.1	1.1
304	1274	12.4	7.8	5.7	45.3	1.8
279	1167	16	6	3	33	1.2
83	352	4	2.7	2	12	0.1
73	310	2	1.5	3	11	0.1
82	345	3	2	3	11	0.1

PIES	AVERAGE PORTION oz	GI	GL
Apple pie, deep filled, double crust	3.8	H	H
Apple pie, double crust	3.8	H	H
Lemon meringue pie	5.3	H	H
Mississippi mud pie	5.3	H	H
Pecan pie	3.5	H	H
Pumpkin pie	3.5	H	H

ICE CREAM AND FROZEN DESSERTS

	AVERAGE PORTION oz	GI	GL
Banana split	3.5	H	H
Chocolate nut sundae	2	H	H
Creamsicle, with fruit coating	2.6	H	H
Frozen ice cream dessert, chocolate	2	H	H
Frozen ice cream dessert, plain	2	H	H
Ice cream, chocolate/caramel	2.8	H	M
Ice cream, dairy-free	2.6	H	M
Ice cream, fruit	2.6	H	M
Ice cream, luxury, vanilla	2.6	H	M
Ice cream, soya	2.6	H	M
Ice cream, vanilla	2.6	H	M
Ice cream, virtually fat-free	2.6	H	M
Ice cream bar, chocolate-covered	2.8	H	M
Ice cream bar, chocolate-flavored coating	1.7	H	M
Ice cream cone, chocolate/chocolate, mint, and nuts	2.5	H	M
Ice cream cone, strawberry	2.9	H	M
Ice cream, soft serve, dairy	2	H	M
Ice cream, soft serve, dairy-free	2	H	M
Popsicle, fruit	2.6	H	H
Peach melba	2	H	H
Sorbet, fruit	2.6	H	H

ENERGY cal	ENERGY J	FAT g	SATURATED FAT g	PROTEIN g	CARBO-HYDRATE g	FIBER g
281	1183	12	3.8	4	42	1.1
269	1129	14	4.5	4	33	1.1
377	1590	13	4.6	4	65	0.7
478	1997	30	15	6	49	3.8
397	1662	18.5	3.5	4	57.2	3.5
203	852	9.5	1.8	3.9	27.3	2.7
182	761	11	6	2	19	0.6
167	699	9	5	2	21	0.1
78	326	2	1	1	15	0.1
150	627	11	8.5	2	13	0
136	568	9	6.7	2	14	Trace
210	880	11.1	7.2	3.4	25.8	0.7
156	654	9	2.8	2	17	0.1
119	499	5	3.4	2	17	0.2
161	670	11	6.8	3	13	0
156	654	9	2.8	2	17	0.1
115	480	6	3.6	2	14	0
76	324	1	Trace	3	15	0
269	1124	16.9	11.4	3.1	27.9	0
142	590	10	8.8	2	11	
204	858	10.1	7.7	2.5	27.7	0.8
201	844	10	7.1	3	28	0.2
101	427	4.9	3.1	1.9	13.2	0
115	484	4.6	3	1.6	17.9	0
56	234	1	0.1	0	14	0.1
98	411	6	3.8	1	10	0.2
98	422	Trace	Trace	1	26	0

CANDY	AVERAGE PORTION oz	GI	GL
Hard candy	0.25	H	H
Coconut/chocolate bar	2	H	H
Chewy candy	0.1	H	H
Chocolate, baking	1.8	M	M
Chocolate, diabetic	1.8	L	M
Chocolate, fancy and filled	0.3	M	M
Chocolate, milk	1.8	M	H
Chocolate, semisweet	1.8	M	M
Chocolate, white	1.8	M	M
Chocolate-covered bar with caramel and cereal	1	M	M
Chocolate-covered bar with fruit/nut	1.2	M	M
Chocolate-covered bar with wafer/cookie	1.2	M	M
Chocolate-covered caramel and biscuit fingers	1	M	M
Chocolate-covered caramels	0.2	M	M
Chocolate-covered cookie fingers	0.9	H	H
Chocolate-covered wafer cookies	0.8	H	H
Creme eggs®	1 .4	H	H
Fruit gums/jellies	0.1	H	H
Fudge	0.4	H	H
M&Ms®-type sweets	0.5	M	M
Marshmallows	0.2	H	H
Nougat	2.5	H	H
Peanut brittle	2	M	M
Peppermints	0.2	H	H
Toffees, mixed	0.3	H	H
Truffles, mocha	0.25	H	H
Truffles, rum	0.25	L	M

ENERGY cal	ENERGY J	FAT g	SATURATED FAT g	PROTEIN g	CARBO-HYDRATE g	FIBER g
23	98	Trace	0	Trace	6	0
270	1129	15	12.1	3	33	1.4
11	48	0.2	0.1	0	2.6	0
275	1147	17	14	2	29	0.6
224	934	15	9.1	5	19	0.6
34	145	1.3	0.8	0.3	5.8	0.2
260	1086	15.6	9.4	3.7	28	0.7
255	1069	14	8.4	3	32	1.3
265	1106	15	9.2	4	29	0
150	631	7.7	4.9	1.6	19.9	0.2
170	711	9	4.6	3	20	1.3
170	711	9	4.6	3	20	1.3
139	582	6.6	3.8	1.4	19.6	0.4
25	103	1.2	0.7	0.2	3.5	0
134	564	7	3.4	2	18	0.3
110	462	6	3.8	2	14	0.2
163	681	6	1.8	2	28	0.5
6	28	0	0	0	2	Trace
49	205	2	1	0	9	0
68	288	3	1.6	1	11	0.2
16	70	0	0	0	4	0
269	1138	6	0.8	3	54	0.6
280	1178	11	3.1	5	43	1.2
24	101	0	0	0	6	0
31	130	1.3	0.7	0.2	5	0
34	143	2	1.1	0	4	0.1
36	152	2	1.4	0	3	0.1

CARBONATED DRINKS

	AVERAGE PORTION fl oz	GI	GL
Club soda	5.6	H	M
Cola	5.6	H	H
Cola, diet	5.6	M	M
Ginger ale, dry	5.6	M	M
Ginger ale, dry, diet	5.6	M	M
Lemonade	5.6	H	H
Lemonade, diet	5.6	M	M
Orangeade	5.6	H	H
Orangeade, diet	5.6	M	M
Root beer	5.6	H	H
Soda, cream	5.6	H	H
Tonic water	5.6	H	M

FRUIT JUICES

	AVERAGE PORTION fl oz	GI	GL
Acai berry	5.6	M	M
Apple, fresh	5.6	M	M
Apple, unsweetened	5.6	M	H
Carrot	5.6	M	M
Grape, unsweetened	5.6	M	M
Grapefruit, unsweetened	5.6	M	M
Lemon, fresh	0.4	M	L
Lime, fresh	0.4	M	L
Mango, canned	5.6	M	M
Orange, fresh	5.6	M	M
Orange, unsweetened	5.6	M	H
Passion fruit	5.6	M	M
Pineapple, unsweetened	5.6	M	M
Pomegranate, fresh	5.6	M	M
Prune	5.6	M	M
Tomato	5.6	M	L
Smoothie made with fruit or fruit juice	10.5	M	M

ENERGY cal	ENERGY J	FAT g	SATURATED FAT g	PROTEIN g	CARBO- HYDRATE g	FIBER g
26	108	0	0	0	6.9	0
66	278	0	0	Trace	17	0
Trace	Trace	0	0	0	0	0
24	99	0	0	0	6	0
2	6	0	0	0	0.4	0
35	149	0	0	Trace	9	0
Trace	Trace	0	0	0	0	0
113	474	0	0	0	27	0
1	4	0	0	0	0.4	0
66	275	0	0	0	17	0
82	344	0	0	0	21	0
53	226	0	0	0	14	0
79	332	0.6	0	0	19.7	0
59	251	0.2	0	0.2	15.5	0
61	262	Trace	Trace	0	16	Trace
38	165	Trace	Trace	1	9	0.2
74	314	Trace	Trace	0	19	0
53	224	Trace	Trace	1	13	Trace
1	3	Trace	Trace	0	0	0
1	4	Trace	Trace	0	0	0
62	266	Trace	Trace	0	16	Trace
54	234	0.2	0	1	13.6	0.3
58	245	Trace	Trace	1	14	0.2
75	302	Trace	Trace	1	17	Trace
66	283	Trace	Trace	0	17	Trace
70	302	Trace	Trace	0	19	Trace
91	389	Trace	Trace	1	23	Trace
22	99	Trace	Trace	1	5	1
188	789	0.4	0.1	1.3	47.9	3

FRUIT SQUASHES AND DRINKS

	AVERAGE PORTION fl. oz	GI	GL
Drink, citrus/apple/mixed fruit flavors	8.8	H	H
Drink, low-calorie, lemon/orange/ mixed fruit flavors	8.8	M	M
Drink, low-sugar, fortified with vitamins	8.8	M	M
Fruit juice drink	7.3	M	M
Fruit juice drink, carbonated	5.6	M	M
Fruit juice drink, low-calorie, mixed fruit flavors	7.3	M	M
High juice drink, orange/lemon flavors	8.8	M	M

MILK-BASED DRINKS

Drinking yogurt	7	M	L
Flavored milk	7.5	H	H
Milkshake, with low-fat milk	10.5	H	H
Milkshake, with skim milk	10.5	H	H
Milkshake, with whole milk	10.5	H	H
Milkshake syrup, with low-fat milk	10.2	H	H
Milkshake syrup, with skim milk	10.2	H	H
Milkshake syrup, with whole milk	10.4	H	H
Probiotic yogurt drink, orange	3.5	M	M
Probiotic yogurt drink, plain	3.5	L	L
Smoothie made with fruit juice and milk/yogurt	10.5	M	M
Soy milk, flavored	5.2	L	L

HOT BEVERAGES

Cappuccino, with low-fat milk	10.2	M	H
Cappuccino, with skim milk	10.2	M	H
Cappuccino, with whole milk	10.2	M	H
Cocoa, with low-fat milk	8.8	M	M
Cocoa, with skim milk	8.8	M	M
Cocoa, with whole milk	8.8	M	M

ENERGY cal	ENERGY J	FAT g	SATURATED FAT g	PROTEIN g	CARBO-HYDRATE g	FIBER g
48	200	0	0	Trace	13	0
3	8	0	0	Trace	1	0
10	43	0	0	Trace	3	0
76	328	Trace	Trace	0	20	Trace
62	264	Trace	Trace	Trace	16	Trace
21	89	Trace	Trace	0	5	Trace
63	268	0	0	0	16	0
124	526	Trace	Trace	6	26	Trace
146	614	3	1.9	8	23	0
207	882	5	3	10	34	Trace
171	726	1	0.3	10	34	0
261	1104	11	7.2	9	33	Trace
171	725	4	2.6	8	27	0
136	576	1	0.2	9	27	0
223	936	10	6.2	8	27	0
67	279	0.9	0.6	1.5	13.4	1.3
68	284	1	0.7	1.7	13.1	1.4
293	1226	4.8	2.8	5.1	61.1	4.5
58	245	2	0.3	4	5	Trace
46	193	2	1	3	5	0
33	141	0	0.1	3	5	0
65	269	4	2.3	3	5	0
143	608	5	3	9	18	0.5
110	475	1	0.8	9	18	0.5
190	800	10	6.5	9	17	0.5

HOT BEVERAGES	AVERAGE PORTION fl oz	GI	GL
Coffee and chicory essence, with water	10.2	L	L
Coffee, drip	10.2	L	L
Coffee, drip, with low-fat milk	10.2	L	L
Coffee, drip, with skim milk	10.2	L	L
Coffee, drip, with single cream	10.2	L	L
Coffee, drip, with whole milk	10.2	L	L
Coffee, instant	10.2	L	L
Coffee, instant, with low-fat milk	10.2	L	L
Coffee, instant, with skim milk	10.2	L	L
Coffee, instant, with whole milk	10.2	L	L
Coffee, Irish	4.4	L	L
Drinking chocolate, with low-fat milk	10.2	H	H
Drinking chocolate, with skim milk	10.2	H	H
Drinking chocolate, with whole milk	10.2	H	H
Latte, with low-fat milk	10.2	L	L
Latte, with skim milk	10.2	L	L
Latte, with whole milk	10.2	L	L
Mocha with low-fat milk	10.2	M	M
Mocha with skim milk	10.2	M	M
Mocha with whole milk	10.2	M	M
Ovaltine, with low-fat milk	10.2	H	H
Ovaltine, with skim milk	10.2	H	H
Ovaltine, with whole milk	10.2	H	H
Tea, black	10.2	L	L
Tea, Chinese	10.2	L	L
Tea, green	10.2	L	L
Tea, herbal	10.2	L	L
Tea, lemon, instant	10.2	M	M
Tea, with low-fat milk	10.2	L	L
Tea with skim milk	10.2	L	L
Tea with whole milk	10.2	L	L

ENERGY cal	ENERGY J	FAT g	SATURATED FAT g	PROTEIN g	CARBO-HYDRATE g	FIBER g
17	76	Trace	0	0	5	0
4	15	Trace	Trace	0	1	0
13	55	1	0.2	1	1	0
11	43	0	0	1	1	0
27	106	2	1.3	1	1	0
13	59	1	0.6	1	1	0
Trace	4	Trace	0	0	Trace	0
13	55	1	0.2	1	1	0
8	39	0	0	1	1	0
15	65	1	0.6	1	1	0
105	433	10	6.1	1	4	0
135	578	4	2.3	7	21	Trace
112	481	1	0.6	7	21	Trace
171	716	8	4.8	6	20	Trace
60	252	2	1.3	4	7	0
33	141	1	0.1	3	5	0
85	353	5	3	4	6	0
96	405	5	3.1	4	9	0.1
81	339	3	2	4	9	0.1
120	500	7	4.8	4	9	0.1
150	642	3	1.9	7	25	Trace
129	549	1	0.2	7	25	Trace
184	779	7	4.6	7	25	Trace
Trace	4	Trace	Trace	0	Trace	0
2	10	0	0	0	0	0
Trace	Trace	0	0	0	Trace	0
2	25	Trace	Trace	0	0	0
15	65	0	0	0	4	0
13	53	1	0.2	1	1	0
8	36	0	0	1	1	0
15	61	1	0.6	1	1	0

ALCOHOLIC DRINKS	AVERAGE PORTION fl oz	GI	GL
Beers			
Bitter, best/premium	10	H	H
Bitter, bottled	10	H	H
Bitter, canned	10	H	H
Bitter, draft	10	H	H
Bitter, keg	10	H	H
Bitter, low-alcohol	8.8	H	H
Brown ale, bottled	8.8	H	H
Mild, draft	10	H	H
Pale ale, bottled	8.8	H	H
Hard ciders			
Dry	10	M	M
Low-alcohol	8.8	M	M
Sweet	10	H	H
Vintage	10	H	H
Lagers			
Bottled	8.8	H	H
Canned	10	H	H
Draft	10	H	H
Low-alcohol	8.8	H	H
Premium	10	H	H
Liqueurs			
Advocaat	0.9	M	M
Campari	1	M	M
Cherry Brandy	0.9	H	H
Coîntreau	0.9	H	H
Cream liqueurs	0.9	H	H
Crème de Menthe	0.9	H	H
Curacao	0.9	H	H
Drambuie	0.9	H	H
Egg nog	5.6	H	H
Grand Marnier	0.9	H	H
Pernod	0.9	H	H
Southern Comfort	0.9	H	H

ENERGY cal	ENERGY J	FAT g	SATURATED FAT g	PROTEIN g	CARBO-HYDRATE g	FIBER g
95	399	Trace	Trace	1	6	Trace
86	356	Trace	Trace	1	6	Trace
92	379	Trace	Trace	1	7	0
92	379	Trace	Trace	1	7	0
89	370	Trace	Trace	1	7	0
33	135	0	0	1	5	Trace
75	315	Trace	Trace	1	8	Trace
69	293	Trace	Trace	1	5	Trace
70	295	Trace	Trace	1	5	Trace
103	436	0	0	Trace	7	0
43	185	0	0	Trace	9	0
121	505	0	0	Trace	12	0
290	1208	0	0	Trace	21	0
73	300	Trace	Trace	1	4	0
83	347	Trace	Trace	1	Trace	Trace
83	347	Trace	Trace	1	Trace	Trace
25	103	Trace	Trace	1	4	Trace
169	700	Trace	Trace	1	7	Trace
65	273	2	0.5	1	7	0
65	272	0	0	0	6.8	0
66	275	0	0	Trace	8	0
79	328	0	0	Trace	6	0
81	338	4	0	Trace	6	0
66	275	0	0	Trace	8	0
78	326	0	0	Trace	7	0
79	328	0	0	Trace	6	0
182	763	7	3.4	6	16	0
79	328	0	0	Trace	6	0
79	328	0	0	Trace	6	0
79	328	0	0	Trace	6	0

ALCOHOLIC DRINKS	AVERAGE PORTION fl oz	GI	GL
Tia Maria	0.9	H	H
Fortified wines			
Port	1.8	M	L
Sherry, dry	1.8	H	L
Sherry, medium	1.8	H	L
Sherry, sweet	1.8	H	L
Vermouth, dry	1.7	H	L
Vermouth, sweet	1.7	H	M
Spirits, 40% volume			
Brandy	0.9	L	L
Gin	0.9	L	L
Rum	0.9	L	L
Vodka	0.9	L	L
Whisky	0.9	L	L
Stout beer			
Bottled	8.8	H	H
Extra	10	H	H
Guinness™	10	H	H
Mackeson	10	H	H
Wines			
Champagne	4.4	L	L
Mulled wine	4.4	L	L
Prosecco	3.5	M	L
Red wine	4.4	L	L
Rose, medium	4.4	L	L
White wine, dry	4.4	L	L
White wine, medium	4.4	L	L
White wine, sparkling	4.4	L	L
White wine, sweet	4.4	L	L
Cocktails			
Daiquiri, canned	1	M	M
Pina colada	1.1	M	M
Tequila sunrise	1.1	M	M
Whiskey sour	1	M	M

ENERGY cal	ENERGY J	FAT g	SATURATED FAT g	PROTEIN g	CARBO- HYDRATE g	FIBER g
66	275	0	0	Trace	8	0
79	328	0	0	0	6	0
58	241	0	0	0	1	0
58	241	0	0	0	3	0
68	284	0	0	0	3	0
52	217	0	0	0	1	0
72	303	0	0	Trace	8	0
52	215	0	0	Trace	Trace	0
52	215	0	0	Trace	Trace	0
52	215	0	0	Trace	Trace	0
52	215	0	0	Trace	Trace	0
52	215	0	0	Trace	Trace	0
93	390	Trace	Trace	1	10	0
112	468	Trace	Trace	1	6	0
86	362	Trace	Trace	1	4	0
103	439	Trace	Trace	1	13	0
95	394	0	0	0	2	0
245	1028	0	0	0	32	0
69	289	0	0	0.1	2	0
85	354	0	0	0	0	0
89	368	0	0	0	3	0
83	344	0	0	0	1	0
93	385	0	0	0	4	0
93	384	0	0	0	6	0
118	493	0	0	0	7	0
38	157	0	0	0	5	0
76	317	2	2.1	0	9	0
35	147	0	0	0	4	0
36	149	0	0	0	4	0

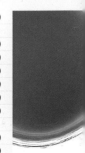
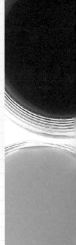

Special Photography
© Octopus Publishing Group Limited/Gareth Sambidge.

Other Photography
© Octopus Publishing Group Limited/Ian O'Leary 8–15, 16–33, 80–85, 86–93, 130–131, 132–143.

Commissioning Editor Nicola Hill
Managing Editor Clare Churly
Design Manager Tokiko Morishima
Designer Peter Gerrish
Picture Librarian Sophie Delpech
Production Assistant Nosheen Shan